GLUTEN-FREE IDEAS

Many Recipes for Your Table to Taste Every Day

ELEANOR FIELDS

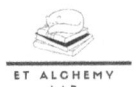
ET ALCHEMY LAB

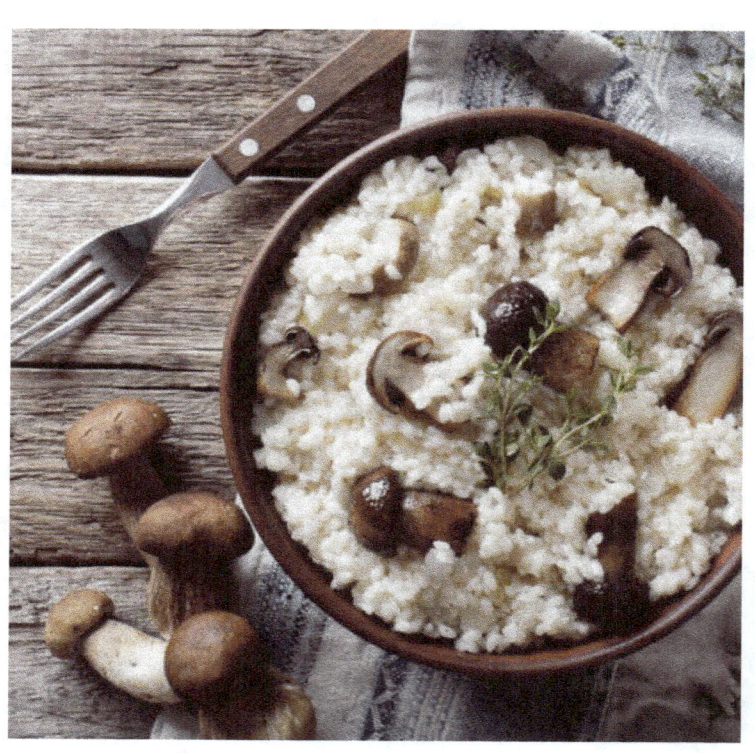

CONTENTS

Introduction	v
1. Celiac Disease	1
2. Substitutions Ideas	7
3. Breakfast	11
4. Lunch	27
5. Dinner	76
6. Snacks and Dessert	114

© Copyright 2021 – Eleanor Fields-All rights reserved.

The content contained within this book may not be reproduced, duplicated or transmitted without direct written permission from the author or the publisher.

Under no circumstances will any blame or legal responsibility be held against the publisher, or author, for any damages, reparation, or monetary loss due to the information contained within this book. Either directly or indirectly.

Legal Notice:

This book is copyright protected. This book is only for personal use. You cannot amend, distribute, sell, use, quote or paraphrase any part, or the content within this book, without the consent of the author or publisher.

Disclaimer Notice:

Please note the information contained within this document is for educational and entertainment purposes only. All effort has been executed to present accurate, up to date, and reliable, complete information. No warranties of any kind are declared or implied. Readers acknowledge that the author is not engaging in the rendering of legal, financial, medical or professional advice. The content within this book has been derived from various sources. Please consult a licensed professional before attempting any techniques outlined in this book.

By reading this document, the reader agrees that under no circumstances is the author responsible for any losses, direct or indirect, which are incurred as a result of the use of information contained within this document, including, but not limited to, — errors, omissions, or inaccuracies.

INTRODUCTION

I never thought I would have a gluten sensitivity. I grew up eating big bowls of pasta on spaghetti night, pizza every Friday, and sugary cereal with my cartoons every morning. In college, I was right there with the rest of my friends, drinking beer, ordering late-night pizza, and never worrying about my weight or how food made my body feel.

But as I entered my twenties and thirties, I started to notice that certain foods would leave me tired, bloated, and not like my best self. Then I had a daughter, and life started to get even busier. Soon I realized that my jeans were a little tighter and my motivation a little lower each day. Just as bad, I felt so tired all the time. It was hard enough to get through my daily to-do list and take care of my family, and I couldn't find the time or energy to go to the gym.

I had heard a lot about gluten and eating gluten-free, but at first, I didn't know if it was necessary for me. That all changed when I talked to some close friends who were all going gluten-free together. They couldn't stop raving about how much better they felt. And when I realized that my friends - who were just as busy and skinny as I was - were suddenly healthier, leaner, and more energetic than I had to do whatever they were doing, and fast.

My husband and I decided to try avoiding gluten in our diet based on the information in a gluten-free book. It changed us. We started thinking about food differently, and we couldn't believe how good it made us feel to avoid just one pesky grain. We felt younger, stronger, and happier than we had in years. But after the first few weeks of our new gluten-free lifestyle, we started missing our favorite foods, like spaghetti and burritos. We needed more variety in our diet, but we didn't want to go back to our old ways, which left us bloated and exhausted after dinner. That's why in this book you will find many ideas to taste your meals as you remember! Hope you will enjoy it!

Chapter One
CELIAC DISEASE

CELIAC DISEASE AND GLUTEN-FREE DIET

Many people who go gluten-free do so because they have celiac disease. The gluten intolerance is an autoimmune disease named Celiac disease in which gluten consumption leads to damage in the small intestine. For those with the disease, their immune system responds to the presence of gluten by launching an attack, which damages vital organs, preventing nutrients from being properly absorbed.

Adults and children show different symptoms, with children more likely to experience digestive issues, including abdominal pain and constipation. Adults may experience fatigue, depression or anxiety, or migraines.

Celiac disease is a hereditary disease so that it can be passed down from generation to generation. Statistics put the chance of developing the celiac disease for someone with a parent, child, or sibling with the disease at 1 in 10.

Currently, the only treatment for celiac disease is an entirely gluten-free diet, but those with they are not the only ones who can eat gluten-free.

Many people who do not have celiac disease still report similar symptoms, such as chronic fatigue, joint pain, and abdominal pain. These people often suffer from what is called non-celiac gluten sensitivity.

While only about 1 in 100 people in the United States are diagnosed with celiac disease, the amount of people who suffer from non-celiac gluten sensitivity is considered much higher. For these people, the ingestion of gluten causes an adverse reaction that is not as extensive as it is for those with celiac disease.

Gluten can also be problematic for those people without a clinical diagnosis of celiac disease. If you or someone you know experiences bloating or inflammation after eating gluten-rich foods like pasta or beer, you don't need to be diagnosed to consider adopting a gluten-free diet.

After all, a gluten-free diet has benefits for everyone, regardless of their gluten tolerance! Cutting out heavy, gluten-laden foods like bread, pasta, and cookies for fresh, light fruits and vegetables is a healthier way to eat for everyone!

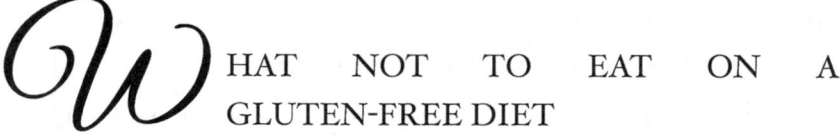HAT NOT TO EAT ON A GLUTEN-FREE DIET

Grains that contain gluten

The big three grains naturally contain gluten are wheat (including Kamut, spelled and triticale), barley, and rye. Other grains and grain products that are not safe for a gluten-free diet because they contain gluten or are at risk of cross-contamination in their production are:

- bran
- bulgur
- couscous
- durum wheat
- flour
- lighthouse
- kamut
- malt
- barley flour or meal
- barley -
- panko
- seitan
- semolina
- udon

Surprising foods that may contain gluten

Unfortunately, gluten has a habit of sneaking into places you wouldn't expect. It's used in all kinds of things that don't seem obvious at first, from chewing gum to shampoo!

Below there is a list of some surprising places where gluten can hide. I've made it as comprehensive as possible, but the best defense against gluten is vigilance! Try to keep an eye on everything you put in your body. Even if you're sure to avoid gluten, it's a good habit to get into.

Alcohol: Depending on the distillation process, some

alcohols may have traces of gluten from the grains they come from.

Baking powder: Make sure you choose one that uses corn or potato starch.

Bleu Cheese: It may have been made with bread mold so that any gluten would be a tiny amount, but you may want to choose a different cheese.

Candy: Yes, even your candy could give you away! A little chocolate with crunchy interiors or caramel coloring may contain gluten, and even a little licorice does!

Canned soup: even unexpected ones like tomato or cream of chicken could hide gluten, so always check the packaging.

Chewing gum: flour may have been used to coat the gum.

Cold cuts: Sometimes contain non-gluten-free components in the form of bread crumbs or sauces.

Flavored potato chips: the chips themselves are usually gluten-free, but not their flavoring powder.

Potato chips: cross-contamination sometimes is dangerous if they are fried in the same fryer as onion rings or other battered or breaded foods.

Sauce: Sauces are typically thickened with flour. Instead, try using cornstarch or arrowroot powder as a thickener at home.

Hot dogs: check the package labels for a gluten-free one.

Ice cream: watch out for cones, and the most dangerous are the types with added ingredients, like cookie dough. Also, make sure the ice cream shop is using a special gluten-free scoop.

Meat imitation: meat substitutes used in sushi or veggie burgers often contain gluten.

Instant coffee and cocoa: instant coffee and cocoa may contain gluten used as a bulking agent.

Meatballs and meatloaf: Both often have breadcrumbs added as a binding agent.

Medications: Gluten is used as a binder in some medications. This can be difficult to discern, but generics are more likely to contain gluten according to experts. before considering any changes related to your medication talk to your doctor.

Mustard: Prepared Mustard

Oatmeal: Oatmeal and oats, in general, should be safe on their own, but they are often contaminated with gluten from the growing and harvesting process. Some brands may be specified as gluten-free, and these are OK.

Omelets: Some restaurant omelets include pancake batter to make them fluffier, so ask before ordering.

Pickles: The pickling process may include malt vinegar, which may contain gluten.

Rice cereal: Rice is OK, but these cereals often contain barley-based flavoring.

Rotisserie Chicken: Not all, but some rotisserie chickens will have added spices that contain gluten. Check the packaging.

Salad dressing: Gluten is often used as a thickener. Be careful with store-bought dressings in general.

Seasoning mixes: read the label before buying any pre-mixed products, as some contain gluten.

Shampoo: You may be thinking, "Well, as long as I can refrain from eating my shampoo, I'll be OK." Unfortunately, what you put on your scalp can get into your body, and shampoos often contain grain-based ingredients. Keep an eye on this and other beauty products, especially if you're celiac or highly reactive to gluten.

Soy sauce: wheat is a key ingredient in soy sauce!

Chapter Two
SUBSTITUTIONS IDEAS

Substitutions that save sanity for your gluten-free pantry While it may seem like pasta, bread, and pizza will be off-limits now that you're gluten-free, once you understand the substitution you can still cook and enjoy many of your favorite recipes s. With the right items in your gluten-free pantry, you'll be able to quickly and easily adapt your cooking to your new healthy life.

However, many gluten-free people find that they tolerate some types of non-grain grains better than others. Some people can eat rice just fine, while others may experience symptoms if they eat it in large quantities. First rule has to be "listen to your body" and experiment with eliminating anything that you feel may be causing you digestive upset.

That is why, the recipes in this book don't rely heavily on gluten-free alternatives or trade other grains for wheat-based products. Many gluten-free people also decide to go grain-free, so I wanted the recipes in this book to work for everyone. Whenever possible, I've suggested various options, both grain-free and non-grain-free, for side dishes, so you'll always have some ideas on what to pair things with.

If you know you can tolerate other types of gluten-free grains, you'll quickly discover that the options for gluten-free alternatives can be overwhelming! Now, almost every grocery store, large and small, carry some gluten-free or gluten-free products. And the great news is: gluten-free products have come a long way. Gone are the days of cardboard-like bread and gummy dough - now you can find delicious, easy-to-use alternatives for everything from pizza crust to dinner rolls to the flour itself.

So, before you feel overwhelmed by all the gluten-free options out there, start with my quick guide to the best gluten-free products. Through much trial and error - and even a few ruined dinners! - I finally found gluten-free alternatives that taste and cook just like the real thing. I hope this was helping you, a few wasted dollars and makes your transition to the gluten-free lifestyle easier and more delicious!

While buying organic produce is not essential to going gluten-free, it is a good way to rid your diet of any traces of pesticides or other chemicals that can also cause inflammation and digestive issues. Buying organic produce can be expensive, but we all want to feed our families healthier and safer fruits and vegetables. That's where Dirty Dozen and Clean Fifteen come in.

The top 15 types of products with the least pesticide residue are known as the Clean Fifteen, while the top 12 most contaminated fruits and vegetables are called the Dirty Dozen.

By knowing which fruits and vegetables contain the most pesticides and which contain the least, you can make more informed choices and stretch your grocery dollar even further.

The Dirty Dozen

Whenever possible, buy these organics:

- Strawberries
- Spinach
- Nectarines
- Apples
- Peaches
- Pears
- Cherries
- Grapes
- Celery
- Tomatoes
- Sweet Peppers
- Potatoes
- Clean Fifteen

The following foods are ok even if they are not organic:

- Corn
- Avocado
- Pineapple
- Cabbage
- Onions

- Sweet Peas
- Papayas
- Asparagus
- Mango
- Eggplant
- Honeydew melon
- Kiwi
- Cantaloupe
- Cauliflower
- Grapefruit

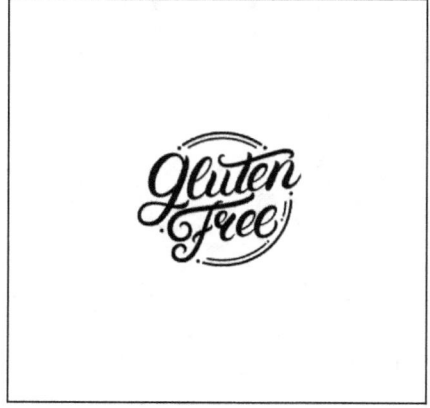

Chapter Three

BREAKFAST

Spinach pancakes

Servings: 4

Ingredients:

- Ghee
- 4 eggs
- 1 pinch of nutmeg
- 70 g chestnut flour

Ingredients:

- 1 pinch of pepper
- 2 handfuls of spinach
- 1/2 teaspoon salt
- 1 handful of rocket

Directions:

- Wash the rocket and spinach. Then puree all the ingredients together.

- Heat some ghee in a pan and fry the dough in portions on both sides.

TOMATO AND SUNFLOWER BREAD

Servings: 1 bread
Ingredients:

- **10 chopped and dried tomatoes**
- **2 tbsp flaxseed flour**
- **1 pinch of rosemary**
- **150 g sunflower seeds**
- **1/2 teaspoon onion powder**
- **100 g pine nuts**

Ingredients:

- 1/2 teaspoon salt
- 2 tbsp ghee
- 2 teaspoons of tartar baking powder
- 1 tbsp tahini
- 4 eggs

Directions:

- First preheat the oven to 180 ° C fan oven. Then grind 120 g sunflower seeds with 40 g pine nuts. Then mix in the remaining seeds.
- Melt the ghee and mix with the flaxseed flour, eggs, tahini, rosemary, baking powder, tomatoes, salt and onion powder. Knead this with the stone mixture. Grease a loaf pan and add the batter.
- Bake it for 40 minutes. Let cool before serving.

PANCAKES WITH RHUBARB COMPOTE

Servings:

Ingredients For the dough:

- **Coconut oil**
- **1 banana**
- **2 tbsp coconut flour**
- **3 eggs**

Ingredients For the compote:

- 1 tbsp honey
- 200 g rhubarb
- 1 vanilla pod
- Juice of one orange

Directions:

- Mash the banana and crack the eggs. Then mix the eggs with the banana and flour. Heat the coconut oil in a pan.
- Bake a quarter of the dough in it. Then process the remaining dough. Wash the rhubarb and cut into small pieces. Scrape the pulp from the vanilla pod.
- Squeeze the orange and bring the juice with the vanilla pulp to the boil. Then reduce the heat and stew the rhubarb in it for 5 minutes.
- Finally stir in the honey. Serve the rhubarb compote with the pancakes.

ALMOND CAPPUCCINO

Servings: 2
Ingredients:

- **1 teaspoon early bird spice**
- **30 g coffee beans**

Ingredients:

- 300 ml almond milk
- 200 ml of water

Directions:

- Grind the coffee beans. Put the water and the powder in an espresso maker and bring to the

boil. Warm the almond milk and fill it into 2 cups.
- Then froth up and pour in the finished espresso.
- Garnish with the seasoning at the end.

SIMPLE KAISERSCHMARRN

Servings: 2
   Ingredients:

- **1 glass of fruit compote**
- **4 eggs**
- **1 pinch of salt**
- **3 tbsp coconut blossom sugar**
- **1 pinch of vanilla**
- **200 ml almond milk**

Ingredients:

- 1 glass of fruit compote
- 4 eggs
- 1 pinch of salt
- 3 tbsp coconut blossom sugar
- 1 pinch of vanilla
- 200 ml almond milk

Directions:

- First separate the eggs. Mix the egg yolks with the

sugar. Then stir in the almond milk and stir in the coconut flour and arrowroot flour.
- Beat the egg whites with a little salt until stiff. Fold the egg whites into the dough. Heat the coconut oil in a pan and bake the dough in it. Then sprinkle with the dried fruit and let it set.
- Pluck the dough into small pieces and finish baking. Finally, serve the Kaiserschmarrn and garnish with cinnamon, vanilla and fruit compote.

CAULIFLOWER PORRIDGE

Servings: 2
Ingredients:

- **Desiccated coconut**
- **1 cauliflower**
- **1 apple**
- **5 tbsp coconut milk**

Ingredients:

- Coconut flakes
- cinnamon
- Pumpkin seeds
- salt

Directions:

- First wash the cauliflower and cut into florets. Boil these in water. Peel, core and cut the apple. Drain the cauliflower.
- Then mix with the coconut milk and the apple pieces. Puree the mixture and season with salt and cinnamon.
- Then fold in the desiccated coconut. Roast the kernels and the coconut flakes without fat and pour them over the porridge.

BREAKFAST CHIPS WITH RASPBERRIES

Servings: 2
Ingredients:

- **2 tbsp coconut oil**
- **1/2 sweet potato**

Ingredients:

- 1 handful of coconut flakes
- 1 handful of raspberries

Directions:

- Heat coconut oil in a pan. Wash and slice the sweet potato.
- Fry these in the pan. Then stir in the coconut flakes and raspberries. Heat everything and serve.

GREEN FRITTATA

Servings:

Ingredients:

- **salt and pepper**
- **1 tbsp coconut milk**
- **6 eggs**

Ingredients:

- 300 g green asparagus
- 2 shallots
- 6 cherry tomatoes

Directions:

- Cut the asparagus into pieces. Wash the cherry tomatoes and cut in half. Peel and chop the shallots. Beat the eggs and whisk together.
- Preheat the oven to 175 ° C. Mix the eggs with the coconut milk and season with salt and pepper.
- Put the vegetables in a mold and pour the eggs on top. Then bake in the oven for 40–45 minutes.

ROASTED ASPARAGUS

Servings:

Ingredients:

- **6 eggs**
- **1 tbsp coconut oil**
- **8 basil leaves**
- **350 g green asparagus**
- **3 teaspoons of dill**

Ingredients:

- salt
- 3 teaspoons of chives
- 1 teaspoon dried oregano
- 1 teaspoon dried rosemary
- 1/2 teaspoon dried marjoram

Directions:

- Wash the asparagus and cut into small pieces. Wash and chop the dill and chives. Whisk the eggs and mix with the chives and dill. Heat the coconut oil in a pan and fry the asparagus in it.
- Then season with salt. Pour the herbs on top and stir. Pour the egg mixture over it and let it set.
- Stir occasionally. Finally, arrange and serve.

SWEET AND SAVORY POTATO PAN

Servings: 2-3
Ingredients:

- **1 tbsp sage**
- **175 g of diced bacon**
- **1 sweet potato**
- **1 onion**

Ingredients:

- 1-2 tbsp coconut oil
- 1 apple
- 1 teaspoon cinnamon

Directions:

- Peel and chop the onion. Wash, peel and dice the apple. Peel and dice the sweet potato. Fry the bacon in a pan. Then remove from the pan and cook the onion, apple and some cinnamon in the same pan.
- Chop the sage. Empty the pan and mix the contents with the bacon. Heat coconut oil again in the same pan. Cook the sweet potato in it.
- Then add the bacon, apple and onion and mix. Stir in the sage before serving.

COLORFUL OMELETTE FROM THE OVEN

Servings: 4-6

Ingredients:

- **salt and pepper**
- **8 eggs**
- **2 teaspoons of chilli flakes**
- **1 broccoli**
- **3 tbsp coconut milk**

Ingredients:

- 1 sweet potato
- 125 g bacon cubes
- 1 bell pepper
- 1 onion

Directions:

- First preheat the oven to 175 ° C. Cut the sweet potato into slices. Grease a baking dish and place the potato slices in it.
- Then season with salt and pepper. Whisk the eggs together and mix in the coconut milk. Season the egg mixture with salt, pepper and the chilli flakes. Peel and chop the onion. Core and dice the peppers.
- Wash the broccoli and cut into florets. Stir this with the onion, bell pepper and bacon into the egg mixture.
- Pour the mixture over the potatoes and cook in the oven for 40 minutes.

SCRAMBLED AVOCADO EGGS WITH SALMON

Servings: 2

Ingredients:

- **salt and pepper**
- **4 eggs**
- **1 teaspoon coconut oil**

Ingredients:

- 100 g smoked salmon
- 1/2 avocado
- 2 tbsp chopped chives

Directions:

- Core the avocado and dice half of the pulp. Whisk the eggs together. Dice the salmon and mix with the eggs.
- Heat the coconut oil in a pan and fry the scrambled eggs in it. Garnish with the avocado and chives. Season again with salt and pepper before serving.

HEARTY BREAKFAST CASSEROLE

Servings: 12

Ingredients:

- **salt and pepper**
- **1 sweet potato**
- **hot paprika powder**

Ingredients:

- 100 g spinach
- 12 eggs
- 2-3 shallots

Directions:

- First preheat the oven to 180 ° C. Dice the sweet potato. Chop the spinach. Peel and chop the shallots as well. Beat the eggs and whisk together.
- Then season the egg mixture with paprika powder, salt and pepper. Grease a baking pan. Put the spinach, onion and sweet potato in a baking pan.
- Pour the egg mixture over it and bake the casserole for 30–35 minutes.

CHIA PUDDING WITH COCOA

Servings: 2

Ingredients:

- **1 tbsp honey**
- **2 cups of coconut milk**
- **1/2 teaspoon cinnamon**

Ingredients:

- 6 tbsp chia seeds
- 1 teaspoon vanilla powder
- 2 teaspoons of cocoa powder

Directions:

- Mix and stir all ingredients. Let the pudding rest in the refrigerator for 60 minutes
- . If you like, you can garnish the pudding with fresh berries.

VEGETABLES BUFFER

Servings: 2-4

Ingredients:

- **Ghee**
- **5 zucchini**
- **1/4 teaspoon cayenne pepper**
- **2 teaspoons of salt**

Ingredients:

- 1 teaspoon pepper
- 1/4 cup coconut flour
- 1 egg

Directions:

- Grate the zucchini and let rest for 10 minutes. Then squeeze out and mix with the egg, coconut flour and pepper. Shape the mixture into buffers
- . Heat the ghee in a pan and fry the buffers on both sides.

CHICORY AND ONION OMELETTE

Servings: 2

Ingredients:

- **salt and pepper**
- **3 chicory**
- **1 tbsp ghee**

Ingredients:

- 4 eggs
- 1/2 bunch of chives
- 1 onion

Directions:

- Wash the chicory and cut in half. Peel and dice the onion. Wash and chop the chives. Heat the ghee in a pan and cook the chicory and onions in it.
- Turn occasionally. Season the chicory. Whisk the

eggs and season with salt and pepper. Pour the egg mixture over the chicory and let it set with the lid closed.
- Then serve the omelette and garnish with chives.

NUT BARS

Servings: 8 bars
Ingredients:

- 3/4 cup dates
- 1 cup of pistachios
- 1/4 cup melted coconut oil
- 1/4 cup pumpkin seeds

Ingredients:

- 1/4 cup hazelnuts
- 3/4 cup desiccated coconut
- 1/4 cup orange juice

Directions:

- Mix the pumpkin seeds with the pistachios, hazelnuts, dates and desiccated coconut. Then mix with coconut oil and the orange juice.
- Lay out the mixture and let it rest for 60 minutes in the refrigerator. Then cut 8 bars out of it and serve.

Chapter Four

LUNCH

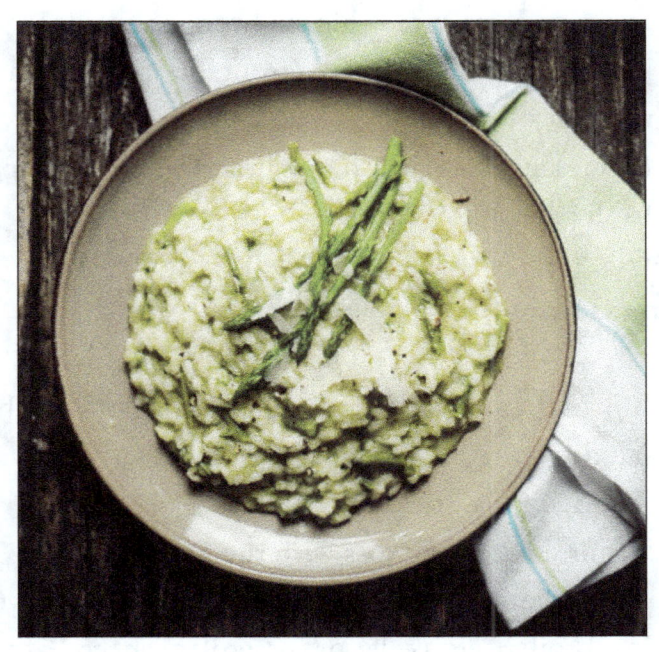

Savory Rice And Sausage

Servings: 4-6

Ingredients:

- 1 pound gluten-free Italian sausage, sweet or hot, cut into 1" pieces
- 1 medium onion, chopped fine
- 2 cloves garlic, chopped
- 1 cup uncooked rice

Ingredients:

- 2¾ cups gluten-free chicken broth
- 1 teaspoon dried rosemary, or 1 tablespoon fresh rosemary
- Parmesan cheese, fresh or gluten-free and chopped fresh parsley, for garnish

Directions:

- Brown the sausage pieces, onion, and garlic. If the sausage is very lean, add a bit of olive oil to prevent the food from sticking.
- Stir in the rice and toss with the sausage and vegetables. Add the broth and rosemary and cover. In a broiler-safe skillet or casserole dish, cook on very low heat or place in a 325°F oven for 45–60

minutes, depending on the type of rice you are using. (Do not use Minute Rice.)
- Just before serving, sprinkle the top with Parmesan cheese and brown under the broiler. Add the chopped parsley and serve.

MEXICAN CHICKEN AND RICE

Servings: 4-6

Ingredients:

- 1/2 cup corn flour
- 1/4 teaspoon salt
- 1/2 teaspoon pepper
- 1 (3 1/2-pound) chicken, cut in serving-sized pieces, rinsed and dried on paper towels
- 1/2 cup corn oil
- 4 cloves garlic, peeled and cut into thick slices
- 1 large red onion, chopped coarsely
- 4 tomatillos, peeled and chopped
- 1 hot pepper, such as serrano or poblano, cored, seeded, and chopped
- 1 sweet red pepper, cored, seeded, and chopped

Ingredients:

- 1/2 cup frozen corn

- 10 mushrooms, chopped
- 1½ cups chopped fresh or canned tomatoes
- 1 cup dry red wine
- 1 lemon, thinly sliced, seeded
- ½ teaspoon cinnamon
- 1 cup short-grained rice, uncooked
- 2 cups gluten-free chicken broth
- ½ cup chopped flat-leaf parsley or cilantro

Directions:

- Mix the corn flour, salt, and pepper on a sheet of wax paper. Dredge the chicken in it.
- Heat the oil in a large frying pan or Dutch oven over medium-high heat. Brown the chicken, for 5–7 minutes. Remove the chicken from the pan and drain on paper towels.
- Add the garlic, onion, tomatillos, hot pepper, sweet pepper, corn, and mushrooms. Sauté until soft, about 10 minutes.
- Add the tomatoes, wine, lemon, and cinnamon. Mix well.
- Return the chicken to the pan and add uncooked rice and broth. Bring to a boil. Then reduce heat to low, cover, and simmer for 45 minutes.
- Just before serving, add the parsley or cilantro. Serve immediately.

HAWAIIAN-STYLE RICE WITH PINEAPPLE, MANGO, AND MACADAMIA NUTS

Servings: 6

Ingredients:

- 1 cup water
- 1½ cups orange juice
- 1½ cups uncooked short-grained rice
- Minced zest of 1 orange
- 1 teaspoon salt

Ingredients:

- 1/8 teaspoon Tabasco sauce
- 1/2 cup chopped pineapple
- 1 ripe mango, peeled and diced
- 2 tablespoons butter
- 1/2 cup toasted macadamia nuts

Directions:

- Bring the water and juice to a boil in a saucepan. Stir in the rice and then add mixture to a greased 2½-quart slow cooker. Cook on high for 2 hours or on low for 4 hours.
- Add the rest of the ingredients on top of the rice

and cook an additional 30 minutes until warmed through.

WILD RICE SALAD WITH RASPBERRY VINAIGRETTE

Servings: 6

Ingredients:

- 4 cups water
- 3/4 cup uncooked wild rice
- 1 teaspoon salt and black pepper, to taste
- 1 small red onion, chopped
- 3 stalks celery, rinsed and chopped finely
- 1 cup water chestnuts, drained and chopped

Ingredients:

- 1 cup jicama, peeled and chopped
- 1 small apple, cored and chopped
- 2/3 cup olive oil
- 1/3 cup raspberry vinegar
- 1/2 cup fresh Italian flat-leaf parsley, rinsed, dried, and chopped
- 6 ounces fresh raspberries, rinsed and set on paper towels to dry

Directions:

- Bring water to a boil and add the rice; return to a rolling boil and then reduce heat to simmer and cover tightly. After 30 minutes, add salt and pepper.
- When the rice has bloomed but is still hot, add the vegetables and apple. Taste and add additional salt and pepper if needed.
- Mix the olive oil and vinegar together with the parsley and combine with the rice and vegetables. Place in a large serving dish and serve warm or chilled. Sprinkle with berries at the last minute.

RISOTTO WITH RADICCHIO AND GORGONZOLA CHEESE

Servings: 4
Ingredients:

- **5 cups gluten-free canned or homemade chicken, fish, or vegetable broth**
- **2 tablespoons butter**
- **2 tablespoons olive oil**
- **½ cup finely chopped sweet onion**
- **1 head radicchio, rinsed and chopped finely**

Ingredients:

- 1½ cups uncooked arborio rice
- Salt and freshly ground black pepper
- ¼ cup crumbled Gorgonzola cheese

- Roasted red pepper strips and chopped parsley, for garnish

Directions:

- Bring the broth to a slow simmer in a saucepan and keep hot.
- Heat the butter and oil in a large, heavy pan; add the onion and radicchio and sauté until softened, about 8 minutes. Add the rice and stir. Add salt and pepper.
- Add the broth, 1/4 cup at a time, until it is all gone, stirring constantly. This will take about 35 minutes. If the risotto is still not done, add water, 1/4 cup at a time.
- When the rice is done, stir in the Gorgonzola cheese and garnish with strips of roasted red pepper and parsley. Serve hot.

PUMPKIN AND BACON RISOTTO

Servings: 4

Ingredients:

- **2 cups fresh pumpkin, peeled, seeded, and diced**
- **Water to cover the pumpkin**
- **1 tablespoon salt**
- **4 strips gluten-free bacon**

- 5 cups gluten-free canned or homemade chicken broth
- 4 tablespoons butter
- ½ cup finely chopped sweet onion

Ingredients:

- 2 teaspoons dried sage or 1 tablespoon chopped fresh
- ½ teaspoon dried oregano or 2 teaspoons chopped fresh
- 1½ cups uncooked arborio rice
- Salt and freshly ground black pepper
- ½ cup Parmesan cheese, fresh or gluten-free
- ¼ cup pepitas, for garnish

Directions:

- Put the diced pumpkin in a saucepan with water to cover and some salt. Simmer until the pumpkin is just tender, drain, and set aside, reserving the pumpkin liquid.
- While the pumpkin is cooking, fry the bacon and drain it on paper towels. Crumble when cool. Heat the chicken broth in a large saucepan and keep at a low simmer.
- Melt the butter in a big, heavy pot and add onion; sauté until soft. Add the sage, oregano, rice, salt, and pepper.

- Slowly add the broth, 1/4 cup at a time. When the pot hisses, add more broth, 1/4 cup at a time. Repeat until broth is gone and then, if still dry, add some of the pumpkin liquid.
- Stir in the pumpkin, Parmesan cheese, and bacon. Add extra pepper or butter if desired. Garnish with a sprinkle of pepitas and serve immediately.

BAKED MUSHROOM AND FONTINA RISOTTO

Servings: 6-8

Ingredients:

- **3 tablespoons butter, divided**
- **3 tablespoons extra-virgin olive oil**
- **1 small onion, minced**
- **2 cloves garlic, minced**
- **1/2 teaspoon salt**
- **1/2 teaspoon pepper**
- **1/2 teaspoon ground oregano**

Ingredients:

- 6 large leaves fresh sage, ripped or cut up, or 2 teaspoons dried sage, crumbled
- 1 cup uncooked long grain rice
- 2 1/2 cups gluten-free chicken broth
- 1/2 cup white vermouth

- 8 ounces mixed mushrooms (shiitake, porcini, morels, chanterelles), sliced
- 1/3 cup grated fontina cheese

Directions:

MOROCCAN HOT AND TASTY WHITE RICE

Servings: 4

Ingredients:

- 3 cups water
- 2 teaspoons salt
- 1 cup uncooked white rice
- 2 cloves garlic, finely minced
- 1 medium onion, finely minced
- 1/2 cup olive oil

Ingredients:

- 6 gluten-free dried apricots, quartered and soaked in 2/3 cup warm water
- 1" harissa (squeezed from tube)—more if you like it really hot. Make sure it's gluten-free.
- 1 teaspoon dried thyme
- Salt, to taste
- 1/2 cup parsley or cilantro, rinsed and chopped

Directions:

- Bring water to a boil and add salt and rice. Reduce heat, cover, and cook until tender, about 25 minutes.
- In a skillet, sauté the garlic and onion in the olive oil over low heat.
- Add the remaining ingredients (including the parsley), and simmer, stirring occasionally, for 10 minutes.
- When the rice is done, mix with the sauce and serve.

CONFETTI AND RICE PASTA WITH CHICKEN

Servings: 4

Ingredients:

- 1/2 cup extra-virgin olive oil
- 1/2 cup finely chopped sweet red pepper
- 1/2 cup finely chopped yellow summer squash
- 1/2 cup zucchini squash, finely chopped
- 1 bunch scallions, chopped fine
- 2 cloves garlic, chopped fine
- 1/2 cup rice or corn flour
- 1 teaspoon salt
- 1/2 teaspoon pepper, or to taste

Ingredients:

- 1/2 teaspoon dried thyme

- ¾ pound boneless, skinless chicken breast, cut into bite-sized pieces
- ½ cup gluten-free chicken broth
- 8 ripe plum (Roma) tomatoes, chopped, or 1½ cups canned
- 1 teaspoon dried oregano
- 1 teaspoon dried basil
- 1 tablespoon red pepper flakes, or to taste
- 1 pound rice pasta, cooked
- 1 cup freshly grated Parmesan cheese

Directions:

- In a large skillet over medium heat, heat the olive oil and add the pepper, squash, scallions, and garlic. Sauté, stirring frequently, for 3–4 minutes.
- While the vegetables are sautéing, mix the flour, salt, pepper, and thyme on a piece of wax paper.
- Dredge the chicken in the flour mixture and add to the pan along with the vegetables.
- Add the broth, tomatoes, oregano, basil, and plenty of red pepper flakes. Cook, uncovered, for 10 minutes to make sure the chicken is done.
- Add the rice pasta to the pan of sauce and mix. Sprinkle with plenty of Parmesan cheese and serve.

PAELLA

Servings: 10-16

Ingredients:

- 2 medium-sized chickens cut into 10 pieces
- 1 pound chorizo (Spanish sausage) or sweet Italian sausage, cut into bite-sized pieces, gluten-free
- 1/2 cup olive oil
- 1 large onion, diced
- 2 cloves garlic, minced
- 3 cups uncooked rice
- 5 1/2 cups gluten-free chicken broth
- **Pinch saffron**

Ingredients:

- 2 tomatoes, cored and chopped
- 1 (10-ounce) box tiny frozen peas (petit pois)
- 18 littleneck clams, scrubbed
- 18 mussels, scrubbed and debearded
- 1 1/2 pounds jumbo shrimp, peeled and deveined
- 1/2 cup chopped fresh parsley

Directions:

- Preheat the oven to 350°F.
- In paella pan or very large skillet, brown the

chicken and chorizo in the olive oil and push them to the side of the pan. Add the onion, garlic, and rice, stirring to soften the onion and garlic and to coat the rice.
- Add the broth, saffron, and tomatoes. Mix well, including the chicken and chorizo.
- Bake in a preheated oven at 350°F for 20 minutes or until the rice begins to take up the broth. Add the peas.
- The order in which you add the seafood is crucial. Always add the ones that take the longest to cook first, adding the more tender pieces at the end. Start by arranging the clams on top. When they start to open, add the mussels. When both are open, add the shrimp and simply mix them into the rice—shrimp take only 2–3 minutes to cook. Sprinkle with parsley and serve in the cooking pan.

LASAGNA WITH SPINACH

Servings: 10

Ingredients:

- 28 ounces low-fat gluten-free ricotta cheese
- 1 cup defrosted and drained frozen cut spinach
- 1 large egg

Ingredients:

- 1/2 cup part-skim shredded mozzarella cheese
- 8 cups (about 2 jars) gluten-free marinara sauce
- 1/2 pound uncooked gluten-free lasagna noodles

Directions:

- In a medium bowl, stir the ricotta, spinach, egg, and mozzarella.
- Ladle a quarter of the marinara sauce along the bottom of a greased 6-quart slow cooker. The bottom should be thoroughly covered in sauce. Add a single layer of lasagna noodles on top of the sauce, breaking noodles if needed to fit in the sides.
- Ladle an additional quarter of sauce over the noodles, covering all of the noodles. Top with half of the cheese mixture, pressing firmly with the back of a spoon to smooth. Add a single layer of lasagna noodles on top of the cheese, breaking noodles if needed to fit in the sides.
- Ladle another quarter of the sauce on top of the noodles, and top with the remaining cheese. Press another layer of noodles onto the cheese and top with the remaining sauce. Take care that the noodles are entirely covered in sauce.
- Cover and cook for 4–6 hours, until cooked through.

EASY ITALIAN SPAGHETTI

Servings: 4

Ingredients:

- 1 pound lean ground beef, browned
- 1 (16-ounce) jar gluten-free marinara sauce
- 1 cup water

Ingredients:

- 8 ounces gluten-free pasta, uncooked
- ½ cup grated Parmesan cheese, fresh or gluten-free

Directions:

- Add browned ground beef, marinara sauce, and water to a greased 4-quart slow cooker.
- Cook on high for 2 hours or on low for 4 hours. About 45 minutes prior to serving, stir dry gluten-free pasta into meat sauce.
- The pasta will cook in the sauce. Serve with Parmesan cheese sprinkled on top of each serving.

CLASSIC ITALIAN RISOTTO

Servings: 4

Ingredients:

- **5 cups gluten-free canned or homemade chicken or vegetable broth**
- **2 tablespoons butter**
- **2 tablespoons extra-virgin olive oil**
- **1/2 cup finely chopped sweet onion**
- **2 stalks celery, finely chopped**
- **1/4 cup celery leaves, chopped**
- **2 cloves garlic, minced**

Ingredients:

- 1 1/2 cups uncooked arborio rice
- 1/3 cup dry white wine
- 1 teaspoon salt, or to taste
- 2/3 cup freshly grated Parmesan cheese
- 1/4 cup chopped parsley
- Freshly ground black pepper, to taste

Directions:

- In a medium saucepan, bring the broth to a slow simmer over low heat and keep it hot.
- Place the butter and oil in a heavy-bottomed pot, melt butter, and add the onion, celery, celery leaves, and garlic. Cook for 8–10 minutes.
- Add the rice and stir to coat with butter and oil. Add white wine and salt.
- In 1/4-cup increments, start adding hot broth. Stir until the broth has been absorbed into the rice.

Add another 1/4 cup, stirring until all of the broth is absorbed. Repeat this process until all of the hot broth is gone. It must be stirred constantly and takes about 35 minutes.
- When all of the broth is gone, taste the rice for desired consistency. If it needs more broth or water, add it and keep stirring. Add the cheese, parsley, and pepper. Serve immediately.

ONE-POT SPAGHETTI AND MEATBALLS

Servings: 4
Ingredients:

- **1 slice gluten-free bread, torn in very small pieces**
- **1/4 cup 2% milk**
- **1 pound lean ground beef**
- **1/2 teaspoon salt**
- **1/2 teaspoon pepper**
- **1 1/2 teaspoons dried onion**

Ingredients:

- 1 large egg
- 1 tablespoon olive oil
- 1 1/2 cups gluten-free prepared spaghetti sauce
- 1/3 cup water
- 4 ounces gluten-free spaghetti, uncooked and

broken into small pieces

Directions:

- In a large bowl, mix together bread and milk. Set aside for 5 minutes. Add ground beef, salt, pepper, dried onion, and egg. Mix well and roll into small meatballs.
- In a skillet over medium heat, cook the meatballs in small batches in the olive oil until they are browned, approximately 5–6 minutes. Add meatballs to a greased 2½-quart slow cooker.
- Add spaghetti sauce and water to the slow cooker. Cook on high for 4 hours or on low for 8 hours.
- An hour before serving, add the spaghetti pieces and stir into the sauce. Cook spaghetti for an hour. Try not to overcook the pasta, as it will become mushy.

GARLIC AND ARTICHOKE PASTA

Servings: 6

Ingredients:

- **2 (14½-ounce) cans diced tomatoes with basil, oregano, and garlic**
- **2 (14-ounce) cans artichoke hearts, drained and quartered**
- **6 cloves garlic, minced**

Ingredients:

- 1/2 cup heavy cream
- 3 cups cooked gluten-free pasta

Directions:

- Pour tomatoes, artichokes, and garlic into a 4-quart slow cooker. Cook on high for 3–4 hours or on low for 6–8 hours.
- Twenty minutes prior to serving, stir in cream.
- Serve over hot gluten-free pasta.

QUINOA WITH CHORIZO

Servings: 4

Ingredients:

- **1/2 cup (or 1 link) Spanish-style chorizo, gluten-free**
- **1/2 cup onions, diced**

Ingredients:

- 1 cup uncooked quinoa, rinsed
- 2 cups water or gluten-free chicken broth

Directions:

- Sauté the chorizo and onions in a small, nonstick skillet over medium heat until the onions are soft. Drain off any excess fat.
- Add to a greased 2½-quart or smaller slow cooker, along with quinoa and water or chicken broth.
- Cover and cook on low for 2 hours or on high for 1 hour, until quinoa is soft and fluffy.

RED RICE AND SAUSAGE

Servings: 4-6

Ingredients:

- **1 pound gluten-free sweet or hot Italian sausage, cut into 1" pieces**
- **1 medium onion, chopped fine**
- **2 cloves garlic, chopped**
- **1 cup red rice, uncooked**

Ingredients:

- 2¾ cups gluten-free chicken broth
- 1 teaspoon dried rosemary or 1 tablespoon fresh rosemary
- ½ cup grated Parmesan cheese, fresh or gluten-free
- ¼ cup chopped fresh parsley

Directions:

- Brown the sausage pieces, onion, and garlic in oven-safe skillet over medium-high heat for 5–8 minutes. If the sausage is very lean, add a bit of olive oil to prevent sticking.
- Stir in the rice and toss with the sausage and vegetables. Add the broth and rosemary and cover. Cook on very low heat or place in a 325°F oven for 45–60 minutes.
- Just before serving, sprinkle the top with Parmesan cheese and brown under the broiler. Add the chopped parsley and serve.

BROWN RICE PILAF WITH TOASTED ALMONDS

Servings: 6

Ingredients:

- 1/3 cup almonds, slivered
- 1 tablespoon extra-virgin olive oil
- 1 large onion, finely chopped
- 3 cloves garlic, minced
- 1 1/2 cups uncooked long grain brown rice

Ingredients:

- 1 teaspoon dried parsley
- 3 1/2 cups gluten-free vegetable broth or low-sodium chicken broth
- 2 teaspoons dried marjoram, minced

- Salt and pepper, to taste

Directions:

- Place the almonds in medium-sized dry skillet over medium heat, stirring constantly for 3–4 minutes, until lightly browned. Place almonds in a small bowl.
- In the same skillet, sauté the onion and garlic in oil. Cook until onion is translucent, about 5 minutes.
- Add the rice and stir until thoroughly mixed, about 1 minute.
- Add parsley, broth, and marjoram; cover and reduce heat to low.
- Simmer until all the water is absorbed and the rice is fully cooked, about 45–50 minutes.
- Uncover, fluff with fork and let stand for a few minutes. Stir in toasted almonds. Add salt and pepper to taste.

ASPARAGUS, MUSHROOMS, AND YELLOW TOMATOES WITH BROWN RICE PASTA

Servings: 6

Ingredients:

- 1 (16-ounce) package of brown rice pasta
- 1 tablespoon extra-virgin olive oil
- 2 cloves garlic, chopped
- 1 pound fresh asparagus, cut in half
- 1 pint yellow tomatoes, sliced in half
- 1 organic yellow pepper, sliced in strips

Ingredients:

- 1 organic orange pepper, sliced in strips
- 1 cup mushrooms, sliced
- ½ cup gluten-free vegetable broth (or broth of your choice)
- 1 tablespoon Parmesan cheese, grated, fresh or gluten-free
- Salt and pepper, to taste

Directions:

- Prepare the brown rice pasta according to the instructions on the package. This pasta should be prepared al dente. Rinse thoroughly with cool water to stop the cooking process and drain.
- Place the oil, garlic, and vegetables in a large skillet and sauté for 3–4 minutes, until they soften. Add

vegetable broth and stir until well blended. Let cook for another 2–3 minutes, until the vegetables are tender.
- Place the vegetables on top of the brown rice pasta and top with freshly shaved Parmesan cheese. Season with salt and pepper to taste if desired.

CORN PASTA IN RICH CREAM SAUCE WITH PROSCIUTTO, GORGONZOLA, AND WALNUTS

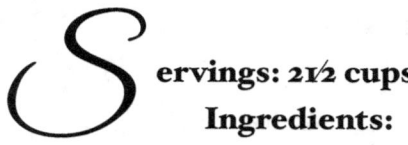

Servings: 2½ cups
Ingredients:

- 1 (10-ounce) package corn pasta
- 3 tablespoons unsalted butter
- 3 tablespoons corn flour
- 2 cups medium cream, warmed
- 2 tablespoons gluten-free minced prosciutto

Ingredients:

- ½ cup crumbled Gorgonzola or blue cheese
- ¼ teaspoon ground nutmeg
- ½ cup walnut pieces, toasted
- Salt and pepper, to taste

Directions:

- Cook corn pasta according to instructions on the package.
- Melt the butter in a large skillet and stir in the flour. Sauté, stirring for 4–5 minutes over medium-low heat. Add the warm cream, whisking constantly until thickened to desired consistency.
- Remove from the heat and stir in the prosciutto, cheese, nutmeg, walnuts, salt, and pepper. Serve immediately.

RICE PASTA IN SPICY SPINACH AND LOBSTER SAUCE

Servings: 4

Ingredients:

- 1 (16-ounce) package rice pasta
- 1 (1½-pound) lobster; if imitation, make sure it is gluten-free
- 2 tablespoons butter
- 2 tablespoons cornstarch
- 1 cup gluten-free hot chicken or clam broth

Ingredients:

- 1 cup heavy cream
- 3 cups fresh baby spinach, rinsed and stems trimmed
- 1 tablespoon dry sherry
- Pinch ground nutmeg
- 1 teaspoon hot red pepper flakes or gluten-free cayenne pepper
- Salt and pepper, to taste

Directions:

- Cook rice pasta according to instructions.
- Plunge the lobster into plenty of boiling salted water. Cook for 15 minutes. Cool; crack the shell and remove the meat. Set the meat aside.
- In a large saucepan, melt the butter and add the cornstarch, stirring until smooth. Whisk in the broth. Add the cream and heat.
- Stir in the spinach and cook until wilted. Add the sherry, nutmeg, red pepper flakes, and reserved lobster. Sprinkle with salt and pepper. Serve over the rice pasta.

ZUCCHINI PASTA WITH PARMESAN AND SPICY MARINARA SAUCE

Servings: 4

Ingredients:

- 4 large zucchini
- 1 tablespoon grapeseed oil
- 2–3 cloves garlic, minced

Ingredients:

- Salt and black pepper, to taste
- 3 tablespoons Parmesan cheese, grated, fresh or gluten-free
- Spicy Marinara Sauce (see recipe in this chapter)

Directions:

- Cut the zucchini into thin, noodle-like strips using a peeler or mandoline.
- Heat the oil in a large skillet over medium-high heat. Add zucchini and garlic; cook and stir until just tender, about 5 minutes. Season to taste with salt and pepper.
- Sprinkle with Parmesan cheese. Top with Spicy Marinara Sauce.

SPICY MARINARA SAUCE

Servings: 10

Ingredients:

- 3 tablespoons extra-virgin olive oil
- 1 medium onion, finely chopped
- 6 cloves garlic, minced
- 1 teaspoon oregano, dried
- 1 teaspoon parsley, dried
- ¾ teaspoon rosemary, dried

Ingredients:

- 1 cup fresh basil leaves, torn
- ¾ teaspoon marjoram
- ½ teaspoon crushed red pepper flakes
- 2 (28-ounce) cans crushed tomatoes
- 1 red bell pepper, seeded and finely chopped
- ½ cup dry white wine
- Salt and pepper, to taste

Directions:

- Heat the olive oil in a large pan. Add onion, garlic, and seasonings. Cover and cook for 10 minutes.
- Add all other ingredients and simmer gently for 75 minutes.

SPRING VEGETABLES WITH PESTO AND PASTA

Servings: 4

Ingredients:

- ½ medium onion, sliced
- 1 tablespoon extra-virgin olive oil
- 1 bunch asparagus, trimmed and cut into 1" pieces
- 3 large carrots, peeled and sliced

Ingredients:

- 1 cup arugula
- ½ cup shelled English peas
- Gluten-free pasta of your choice
- Classic Pesto Sauce

Directions:

- Place the onion in a large skillet with oil. Sauté for 3–4 minutes, until translucent.
- Add asparagus and carrots. Cook for 5 minutes, until their colors brighten and they become tender.
- Add arugula and peas, and stir to combine for 1 minute until arugula wilts. Remove from heat and place in a large bowl.
- Cook pasta according to instructions. When

finished cooking, toss vegetables and pasta together. Add the amount of pesto to your liking.

QUINOA ANGEL HAIR WITH BOLOGNESE SAUCE

Servings: 4-6

Ingredients:

- 1 tablespoon extra-virgin olive oil
- 2 cloves garlic, chopped
- 1/2 medium onion, chopped
- 1 pound lean ground beef, turkey, or chicken
- 2 ounces gluten-free diced pancetta
- 1/2 cup lean ground pork

Ingredients:

- 1/2 cup chopped mushrooms
- 1/2 cup chopped carrots
- Spicy Marinara Sauce (see recipe in this chapter)
- 1 (8-ounce) package quinoa angel hair pasta
- Parmesan cheese, for topping (optional), fresh or gluten-free

Directions:

- In a large skillet over medium heat, place the oil, garlic, and onion. Sauté for 3–4 minutes, until onions are translucent and tender.

- Add the ground beef, pancetta, and ground pork and brown over medium heat until no longer pink, about 5–8 minutes.
- Once the meat is cooked, add mushrooms and carrots and cook for 3–4 minutes, until they soften.
- Add Spicy Marinara Sauce (you can adjust the spices, when preparing the Spicy Marinara Sauce, according to your tastes) and let simmer over low heat for 20–25 minutes, stirring occasionally.
- Cook quinoa angel hair according to instructions. Place Bolognese sauce on top. Add grated Parmesan cheese if desired.

PASTA PRIMAVERA WITH SUMMER VEGETABLES

Servings: 6

Ingredients:

- 16 ounces gluten-free pasta of your choice
- 3 tablespoons extra-virgin olive oil
- ½ green onion, chopped
- 2 cloves garlic, minced
- 1 large carrot, peeled and diced
- 1 large zucchini, peeled and diced
- 1 summer squash, peeled and diced
- ½ medium green bell pepper, seeded and diced

Ingredients:

- ½ medium red bell pepper, seeded and diced
- ½ cup chopped green beans
- ½ small eggplant, peeled and cut crosswise into ¼" slices
- ½ cup sliced plum (Roma) tomatoes
- ½ cup Spicy Marinara Sauce (see recipe in this chapter)
- Grated Parmesan cheese, fresh or gluten-free, for topping (optional)
- Salt and pepper, to taste

Directions:

- Cook pasta according to package instructions. Rinse with cool water and set aside.
- In a large skillet over medium heat, add the oil, onion, and garlic. Cook for 2–3 minutes, until onions and garlic become tender.
- Add the vegetables and stir to combine. Cook vegetables about 10 minutes, until they soften. Remove from heat.
- Add the marinara sauce to the vegetables and stir to combine. Add pasta and stir once again. Top with grated Parmesan cheese and salt and pepper to taste.

BROWN RICE WITH BABY SPINACH, TOMATOES, AND GRILLED TURKEY SAUSAGE

Servings: 6

Ingredients:

- 1 1/2 cups brown rice, uncooked
- 1 (16-ounce) package turkey sausage, gluten-free
- 1/4 teaspoon grapeseed oil
- 2 cloves garlic, chopped
- 2 cups organic baby spinach
- 1/2 pint grape or cherry tomatoes, sliced in half

Ingredients:

- 1 yellow pepper, cut in 1" slices
- 1/4 cup gluten-free chicken broth
- 1/2 teaspoon sea salt
- Pepper, to taste
- 1/2 teaspoon oregano
- 1 tablespoon fresh basil, torn

Directions:

- Cook rice according to instructions.

- Grill sausage in a grill pan or on the grill for 5–8 minutes, until browned and no longer pink. Set aside.
- In a saucepan over medium heat, place oil and garlic, and sauté for 1–2 minutes, until garlic softens.
- Add the spinach, tomatoes, and pepper and cook for 3–4 minutes, until vegetables are tender.
- Add the chicken broth, salt, pepper, and oregano, turn heat to low, and let simmer for 3–4 more minutes.
- Add cooked sausage and stir to combine. Pour sausage/vegetable mixture over rice and serve immediately. Top with fresh basil.

PERSIAN RICE WITH SAFFRON AND SOUR CHERRIES

Servings: 6-8

Ingredients:

- **1 tablespoon extra-virgin olive oil**
- **1½ cups uncooked basmati or other long-grain rice**
- **2½ cups gluten-free chicken broth**
- **1 teaspoon saffron threads**
- **1 (8-ounce) jar imported Iranian sour cherries, blanched, with juice**

Ingredients:

- 1 tablespoon butter
- 1 teaspoon salt
- Freshly ground pepper, to taste
- 1/2 cup slivered almonds, toasted, for garnish

Directions:

- Heat the oil in a large skillet and add the rice; cook, stirring, for 6 minutes.
- Add the chicken broth and bring to a boil. Reduce heat to low and add all remaining ingredients, except the almonds.
- Cover and simmer for 25 minutes, or until the rice is tender. Check the rice every 10 minutes to make sure it does not dry out. If the rice is stubbornly tough, add more broth, or water.
- Place in a warm serving bowl and sprinkle with almonds.

BEEF-FLAVORED WHITE RICE WITH ASIAN SPICES

Servings: 4

Ingredients:

- 1/2 cup gluten-free soy sauce
- 1/4 cup dry white wine or sake
- 1 tablespoon freshly grated gingerroot
- 1 tablespoon Asian sesame seed oil

- **1 teaspoon gluten-free Asian five-spice powder**

Ingredients:

- 2 cloves garlic, minced
- 4 scallions, minced
- ⅔ cup gluten-free beef broth
- 3 cups hot, cooked white rice

Directions:

- Mix together all ingredients, except the rice, to make a sauce.
- Boil for 3 minutes to reduce.
- Then mix in the rice, and serve hot.

SPANISH-STYLE RICE

Servings: 4

Ingredients:

- **3 cups water**
- **2 teaspoons salt**
- **1 cup white rice, uncooked**
- **½ cup extra-virgin olive oil**
- **1 large onion, chopped**
- **1 clove garlic**
- **½ teaspoon oregano, dried**

Ingredients:

- 2 jalapeño or poblano peppers, cored, seeded, and chopped
- 1 roasted red pepper, from a jar or your own, chopped
- 4 ripe plum (Roma) tomatoes, cored and chopped
- 1 teaspoon lemon zest
- 10 black olives, sliced
- Freshly ground black pepper, to taste

Directions:

- In a large saucepan, bring the water to a boil, and add the salt and the rice. Reduce the heat to low, cover, and simmer until tender, about 25 minutes.
- While the rice is cooking, heat the oil in a large frying pan.
- Add the onion, garlic, oregano, and hot peppers. Sauté over low flame for 8–10 minutes.
- Mix in the rest of the ingredients and simmer for 10 minutes.
- Add to the hot rice and serve.

RANGOON RICE CAKES

Servings: 6

Ingredients:

- **6 cups cooked rice**
- **1/2 cup minced red onion**
- **1 clove garlic, chopped**
- **1" fresh gingerroot, peeled and minced**
- **1 tablespoon gluten-free madras curry powder**
- **1/2 teaspoon cinnamon**
- **2 large eggs**
- **1/2 cup heavy cream**

Ingredients:

- 1 teaspoon salt and black pepper, to taste
- 1/4–1/2 cup cooking oil, as needed
- 2 cups gluten-free bread crumbs
- 1/2 cucumber, chopped
- 1/2 cup plain gluten-free yogurt
- Juice of 1/2 lemon
- 12 mint leaves, for garnish

Directions:

- In a large bowl, mix the rice, onion, garlic, gingerroot, and spices together.
- Add the eggs and cream and keep mixing. Sprinkle with salt and pepper to taste and combine well.
- Form into 12 small cakes. (The recipe can be made up to this point in advance and refrigerated for up to a day.)

- Heat oil in a frying pan over high heat. Cover the cakes with crumbs and fry until golden. Place on paper towels to drain, and then on a warm platter.
- Mix chopped cucumber, yogurt, and lemon. Place in a bowl on the side of the dish of rice balls. Serve rice balls with a mint leaf on top of each cake.

WILD RICE STUFFING FOR POULTRY

Servings: makes enough stuffing for a 12-pound turkey
Ingredients:

- **1/4 pound butter**
- **1 large onion, chopped**
- **3 stalks celery with their tops, rinsed and chopped**
- **1 teaspoon each: dried thyme, dried rosemary, dried sage, salt, and pepper**
- **1 cup walnut halves, toasted and chopped**

Ingredients:

- 3 tart apples, peeled, cored, and chopped
- 1/2 cup dry white wine
- 1/2 cup fresh parsley, rinsed and chopped
- 6 cups cooked wild rice

Directions:

- In a large skillet, melt the butter and add onion, celery, herbs, salt, and pepper. Sauté until vegetables are softened, about 5 minutes. Add the walnuts and apples as well as wine and parsley.
- Mix all of the ingredients in a large bowl, tossing with the wild rice until well combined.
- Either stuff it into the turkey or spoon it into a casserole dish and bake at 350°F for 30 minutes, covered with aluminum foil.

CORN TORTILLA CASSEROLE

Servings: 8

Ingredients:

- 2 tablespoons olive oil
- 2 pounds lean ground beef
- 1 small onion, peeled and diced
- 1 clove garlic, minced
- 1 envelope gluten-free taco seasoning
- 1/2 teaspoon salt
- 1/2 teaspoon freshly ground pepper

Ingredients:

- 1 (15-ounce) can diced tomatoes
- 1 (6-ounce) can tomato paste
- 2 cups refried beans
- 9 gluten-free corn tortillas

- 2 cups gluten-free enchilada sauce
- 2 cups (8 ounces) grated Cheddar cheese

Directions:

- In a large skillet, heat olive oil. Brown ground beef for approximately 5–6 minutes and set aside in a large bowl. In the same skillet, sauté onions until softened, about 3–5 minutes. Add sautéed onions to ground beef.
- Stir in the garlic, taco seasoning, salt, pepper, tomatoes, tomato paste, and refried beans into the ground beef and onions.
- Grease a 4-quart slow cooker with nonstick spray. Add 1/3 of the ground beef mixture to cover the bottom of the slow cooker insert. Layer 3 tortillas on top of the ground beef mixture and cover with 1/3 of the enchilada sauce, then 1/3 of the shredded cheese. Repeat layers. Cover and cook on low for 6–8 hours. Cut into 8 wedges and serve.

STUFFED FILET MIGNON WITH RED WINE SAUCE

Servings: 10-12

Ingredients:

- **4 tablespoons unsalted butter**
- **4 cups exotic mushrooms such as creminis,**

morels, shiitake, or oysters, brushed off, stems removed, chopped finely
- 6 shallots, peeled and minced
- 4 cloves garlic, peeled and minced
- 1 tablespoon gluten-free Worcestershire sauce
- 1/4 cup chestnut flour, mixed with salt and pepper, to taste
- 1/2 cup dry red wine, divided
- 4 sage leaves, torn in small pieces

Ingredients:

- 1/2 teaspoon dried rosemary
- 1/2 teaspoon dried thyme
- 1 (6-pound) filet mignon, fat trimmed
- 1/2 cup chestnut flour
- 1 tablespoon coarse salt
- 1 teaspoon black pepper
- 1 cup gluten-free beef broth
- 2 tablespoons extra-virgin olive oil

Directions:

- In a large skillet over medium heat, melt the butter. Add the mushrooms, shallots, and garlic, and sauté until the vegetables are soft and the mushrooms are wilted, about 3–4 minutes.
- Add the Worcestershire sauce. Add 1/4 cup flour

seasoned with salt and pepper and blend. Stir in red wine and the sage, rosemary, and thyme. Reduce the mixture to about 1½ cups, about 5–7 minutes.
- Preheat oven to 350°F.
- Make a tunnel down the middle of the filet mignon—use a fat knitting needle or the handle of a blunt knife. Stuff the mushroom mixture into the tube. If there are extra mushrooms, save them for the sauce.
- Coat the outside of the filet with ½ cup chestnut flour, salt, and pepper. Place the beef broth in the bottom of a roasting pan with the filet. Sprinkle with olive oil and roast in oven for 20 minutes per pound.

MARINATED SPICY BEEF AND BABY SPINACH

Servings: 4
   Ingredients:

- 2 cloves garlic, minced
- 2 tablespoons sugar
- ½ teaspoon salt, or to taste
- 1 teaspoon red pepper flakes, or to taste
- 2 tablespoons canola oil
- 1½ pounds filet mignon, trimmed and cut into ½" slices
- ¼ cup dry white wine

Ingredients:

- 1/4 cup white wine vinegar (not malt)
- 2 teaspoons sugar
- 2 tablespoons gluten-free fish sauce
- 2 tablespoons canola or peanut oil
- 4 cups fresh baby spinach, rinsed, spun dry, stems removed
- 1 tablespoon butter
- Gluten-free soy sauce, chopped scallions, and lemon and lime slices, for garnish

Directions:

- In a large bowl or glass baking dish, mix together the garlic, 2 tablespoons sugar, salt, pepper flakes, and 2 tablespoons oil. Add the slices of filet mignon, turning to coat. Cover and refrigerate for 2 hours.
- Mix together the wine, vinegar, 2 teaspoons sugar, and fish sauce; set aside. Heat a nonstick pan over very high heat and add 2 tablespoons oil. Quickly sauté the filets until browned on both sides, about 2 minutes per side. Arrange the meat over a bed of spinach.
- Add the wine mixture and butter to the pan and deglaze, reducing quickly. Pour over the spinach and meat. Serve with gluten-free soy sauce and

chopped scallions on the side and slices of lemon or lime.

GASCONY-STYLE POT ROAST

Servings: 6

Ingredients:

- 1 (4-pound) top or bottom round beef roast
- 4 cloves garlic, slivered
- 1 teaspoon salt
- 1 teaspoon freshly ground black pepper
- Pinch each of cinnamon and nutmeg
- 1 slice gluten-free bacon, cut into pieces
- 4 shallots, peeled and halved

Ingredients:

- 2 red onions, peeled and quartered
- 2 ounces cognac
- 2 cups red wine
- 1 cup rich gluten-free beef broth
- 1 teaspoon thyme
- 4 whole cloves
- 1/4 cup cornstarch mixed with 1/3 cup cold water until smooth

Directions:

- Make several cuts in the meat and put slivers of garlic in each. Rub the roast with salt, pepper, and pinches of cinnamon and nutmeg.
- Heat the bacon on the bottom of a Dutch oven. Remove the bacon before it gets crisp, and brown the roast. Surround the roast with shallots and onions. Add the cognac, wine, beef broth, thyme, and cloves.
- Place in a 250°F oven for 5–6 hours. When the meat is done, place the roast on a warm platter. Add the cornstarch-and-water mixture to the pan juices and bring to a boil. Slice the roast. Serve the sauce over the pot roast with the vegetables surrounding the meat.

STUFFED, ROASTED FILET MIGNON

Servings: 10-12

Ingredients:

- 1 pound fresh spinach, washed, cut up, blanched, and squeezed to remove extra moisture, or 2 (10-ounce) boxes frozen spinach, thawed and drained
- 2 tablespoons olive oil
- 4 cloves garlic, minced
- Juice of 1/2 lemon
- 1/4 teaspoon nutmeg

Ingredients:

- 1 cup gluten-free soft bread crumbs mixed with seasonings such as dried oregano and salt and pepper, to taste
- 1 (6-pound) filet mignon, well trimmed
- 1 teaspoon salt and freshly ground black pepper, to taste
- 2 tablespoons softened butter
- 1 (13-ounce) can gluten-free low-salt beef broth

Directions:

- Preheat the oven to 350°F.
- Place the spinach on paper towels to dry a bit. Heat the olive oil in a medium-sized fry pan and add the garlic; cook over medium heat to soften. Stirring, mix in the spinach, lemon juice, and nutmeg. Add the bread crumbs.
- Using a fat knitting needle or the handle of a dull knife, make a channel through the meat. Force in the stuffing.
- Sprinkle the meat with salt and pepper, then rub with the softened butter. Roast in oven for 60 minutes, basting every 15 minutes with the beef broth. Reserve pan juice for another use. Let the filet rest for 15 minutes before serving.

Chapter Five

DINNER

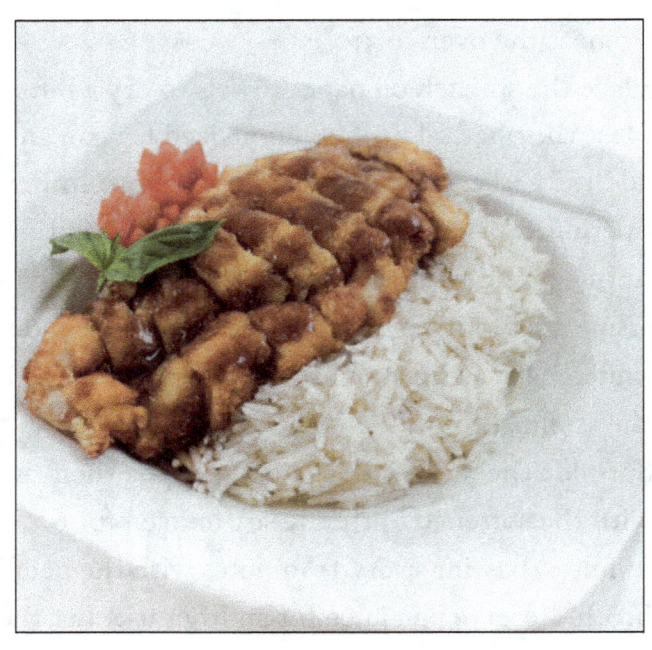

Lentil Salad

Servings: 6

Ingredients:

- 1 (16-ounce) package red lentils or small French ones
- 2 cups gluten-free chicken broth
- Water, as needed
- 2 cloves garlic, smashed and peeled
- 2 whole cloves
- 4 slices gluten-free smoked bacon
- 1/2 cup finely chopped sweet red onion
- 1 sweet red bell pepper, roasted, peeled, and chopped
- 2 stalks celery, washed and finely chopped

Ingredients:

- 1/2 cup chopped fresh parsley
- 2 teaspoons dried oregano
- 1 teaspoon prepared gluten-free Dijon mustard
- 2 tablespoons lemon juice
- 2 tablespoons red wine vinegar
- 2/3 cup extra-virgin olive oil
- Salt and freshly ground pepper, to taste

Directions:

- In a large saucepan, combine the lentils and broth, and add water to cover. Add the garlic and cloves. Bring the lentils to a boil and reduce heat to simmer. Cook until tender, about 20 minutes. Drain and place in a large serving bowl. Remove garlic and cloves.
- Cook bacon, and drain on paper towels.
- Mix the rest of the ingredients with the lentils and chill for 2–3 hours. Just before serving, heat for a few seconds in the microwave. Or serve well chilled with shredded lettuce. Garnish with crisp chopped bacon.

TUSCAN BEAN, TOMATO, AND PARMESAN CASSEROLE

Servings: 4-6

Ingredients:

- 4 slices gluten-free bacon
- 1/4 cup extra-virgin olive oil
- 4 cloves garlic, chopped coarsely
- 1 medium onion, peeled and chopped coarsely
- 1/2 fresh fennel bulb, coarsely chopped
- 1 tablespoon rice flour
- 2 (15-ounce) cans white beans, drained and rinsed
- 16 ounces tomatoes, chopped (canned is fine)

Ingredients:

- 1 medium zucchini, chopped
- 1 tablespoon chopped fresh basil
- 1 teaspoon dried oregano
- 1 teaspoon dried rosemary
- 1/2 cup fresh Italian parsley, rinsed and chopped
- 1 teaspoon dried red pepper flakes, or to taste
- 1 teaspoon salt, or to taste
- 1/2 cup freshly grated Parmesan cheese, fresh or gluten-free
- 2 tablespoons unsalted butter, cut into small pieces

Directions:

- Preheat oven to 350°F.
- Fry the bacon in a skillet until almost crisp. Place on paper towels to drain. Remove all but 1 teaspoon of bacon fat from pan. Chop bacon and set aside.
- Add the oil, garlic, onion, and fennel to the skillet. Sauté over low heat for 10 minutes, or until softened but not browned.
- Blend the flour into the mixture and cook for 3 minutes, mixing well.
- Add the beans, tomatoes, and zucchini. Mix well and pour into a casserole dish.
- Add the herbs, red pepper flakes, and salt, and stir. Mix in the reserved chopped bacon.

- Sprinkle Parmesan cheese and butter over the top and bake for 25 minutes, or until the cheese is lightly browned.

INDIAN-STYLE CHICKEN WITH LENTILS

Servings: 4-6

Ingredients:

- 1 cup uncooked lentils
- 3 cups water
- Salt and red pepper flakes, to taste
- 2 cloves garlic, peeled and minced
- 1 medium onion, peeled and finely minced
- 2 tablespoons lemon juice

Ingredients:

- 1 teaspoon cumin
- 1/2 cup chopped fresh parsley
- 1 pound boneless, skinless chicken breasts, cut into bite-sized pieces
- 1 cup plain gluten-free yogurt
- 1 tablespoon gluten-free curry powder
- Salt and Tabasco sauce, to taste

Directions:

- Place the lentils and water in a saucepan. Bring to a boil, reduce heat, and simmer.
- Just before the lentils are cooked (when barely tender, after about 25 minutes), add the salt and pepper flakes, garlic, onion, lemon juice, cumin, and parsley until the onion is soft and lentils are finished cooking.
- Toss the chicken with the yogurt, curry powder, salt, and Tabasco. Place on aluminum foil and broil for 5 minutes per side.
- Mix the chicken into the lentils and serve with rice.

THICK AND CREAMY CORN AND LIMA BEAN CASSEROLE

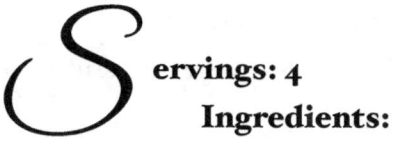

Servings: 4

Ingredients:

- 2 tablespoons butter
- 1/2 sweet onion, finely chopped
- 1/2 cup minced celery
- 1/4 cup minced roasted red pepper
- 1/2 cup gluten-free chicken broth
- 1 (10-ounce) package frozen lima beans

- 1 (10-ounce) package frozen corn kernels

Ingredients:

- 2 large eggs, well beaten
- 1½ cups heavy cream or evaporated milk
- 1 teaspoon salt
- 1 teaspoon paprika
- 1 teaspoon ground black pepper
- 1 teaspoon ground coriander
- ½ teaspoon ground allspice
- 1 cup gluten-free bread crumbs

Directions:

- Melt butter in a large skillet. Sauté onion and celery until softened, about 3–5 minutes.
- Grease a 4-quart slow cooker. Add sautéed onions and celery. Add remaining ingredients to slow cooker, except for bread crumbs. Stir together and sprinkle bread crumbs on top.
- Cover and vent the lid with a chopstick. Cook on low for 6 hours or on high for 3 hours.

RED BEANS AND RICE

Servings: 6

Ingredients:

- 1 tablespoon olive oil
- 1 cup converted long-grain rice, uncooked
- 1 (15-ounce) can red beans, rinsed and drained
- 1 (15-ounce) can pinto beans, rinsed and drained
- ½ teaspoon salt

Ingredients:

- 1 teaspoon gluten-free Italian seasoning
- ½ tablespoon dried onion flakes
- 1 (15-ounce) can diced tomatoes
- 1¼ cups gluten-free vegetable broth or water

Directions:

- Grease a 4-quart slow cooker with nonstick spray. Add the oil and rice; stir to coat the rice in the oil.
- Add the red beans, pinto beans, salt, Italian seasoning, onion flakes, tomatoes, and vegetable broth or water to the slow cooker. Stir to combine. Cover and cook on low for 6 hours or until the rice is tender.

WHITE BEAN CASSOULET

Servings: 8
Ingredients:

- **1 pound dried cannellini beans**
- **2 leeks, sliced**
- **1 teaspoon canola oil**
- **2 parsnips, diced**
- **2 carrots, diced**
- **2 stalks celery, diced**
- **1 cup sliced baby bella mushrooms**

Ingredients:

- 1/2 teaspoon ground fennel
- 1 teaspoon crushed rosemary
- 1 teaspoon dried parsley
- 1/8 teaspoon ground cloves
- 1/4 teaspoon salt
- 1/4 teaspoon freshly ground black pepper
- 2 cups gluten-free vegetable broth

Directions:

- The night before making the soup, place the beans in a 4-quart slow cooker. Fill with water to 1" below the top of the insert. Soak overnight.
- Drain and rinse the beans and return them to the slow cooker.
- Slice only the white and light-green parts of the leeks into 1/4" rounds. Cut the rounds in half.
- Heat the oil in a nonstick skillet. Add the parsnips, carrots, celery, mushrooms, and sliced leeks. Sauté

for 1 minute, just until the color of the vegetables brightens. Add vegetables to the slow cooker along with the broth, herbs, and spices.
- Cook on low for 8–10 hours.

SLOW-COOKED SOUTHERN LIMA BEANS WITH HAM

Servings: 8

Ingredients:

- **1 pound dry lima beans, soaked for 6–8 hours and rinsed with cold water**
- **2 cups gluten-free cooked ham, diced**
- **1 sweet onion, chopped**
- **1 teaspoon dry mustard**

Ingredients:

- 1 teaspoon salt
- 1/2 teaspoon freshly ground pepper
- 2 cups water
- 1 (15 1/2-ounce) can tomato sauce

Directions:

- Drain and rinse soaked lima beans. Add beans to a greased 4–6-quart slow cooker. Add all remaining ingredients. If needed add additional water to cover the beans by 1".

- Cook on high for 4 hours or on low for 8 hours. Serve over cooked rice or gluten-free pasta.

CURRIED LENTILS

Servings: 6

Ingredients:

- 2 teaspoons canola oil
- 1 large onion, thinly sliced
- 2 cloves garlic, minced
- 2 jalapeños, seeded and diced
- 1/2 teaspoon red pepper flakes
- 1/2 teaspoon ground cumin

Ingredients:

- 1 pound uncooked yellow lentils
- 6 cups water
- 1/2 teaspoon salt
- 1/2 teaspoon ground turmeric
- 4 cups chopped fresh spinach

Directions:

- Heat the oil in a nonstick pan. Sauté the onion slices until they start to brown, about 8–10 minutes.
- Add the garlic, jalapeños, red pepper flakes, and

cumin. Sauté for 2–3 minutes. Add the onion mixture to a 4-quart slow cooker.
- Sort through the lentils and discard any rocks or foreign matter. Add the lentils to the slow cooker.
- Add the water, salt, and turmeric to the slow cooker and stir to combine. Cook on high for 2½ hours.
- Add the spinach. Stir and cook on high for an additional 15 minutes.

EASY REFRIED BEANS

Servings: 8

Ingredients:

- 3 cups dried pinto beans
- 1 large onion, peeled and halved
- ½ fresh jalapeño pepper, seeded and chopped
- 6 cloves garlic, peeled and minced

Ingredients:

- ⅛ teaspoon ground cumin
- 9 cups water
- 1 teaspoon salt
- ½ teaspoon freshly ground black pepper

Directions:

- Rinse and drain beans and place them in a bowl or saucepan. Add enough water to cover the beans by 2 inches. Cover and let soak overnight or for 8 hours. Drain the beans, then rinse and drain again.
- Add the soaked beans, onion, jalapeño, garlic, and cumin to a 6-quart slow cooker. Pour in the water and stir to combine. Cover and, stirring occasionally, and adding more water as needed, cook on high for 8 hours or until the beans are cooked through and tender. (If you have to add more than 1 cup of water during cooking, lower the temperature to low or simmer.)
- Once the beans are cooked, strain them, reserving the liquid. Mash the beans with a potato masher, adding some of the reserved water as needed to attain desired consistency. Add salt and pepper.

BEANS GALORE

Servings: 8

Ingredients:

- ½ pound gluten-free bacon
- 1 pound lean ground beef
- 1 medium onion, chopped
- ¼ cup brown sugar
- ¼ cup white sugar
- ¼ cup gluten-free ketchup
- ¼ cup gluten-free barbecue sauce

Ingredients:

- 1 teaspoon dry mustard
- 2 tablespoons molasses
- 1/2 teaspoon gluten-free chili powder
- 1/2 teaspoon ground pepper
- 1 teaspoon salt
- 2 (15-ounce) cans gluten-free pork and beans (do not drain)
- 1 (15-ounce) can red kidney beans (do not drain)
- 1 (15-ounce) can lima beans (do not drain)

Directions:

- Fry bacon in a skillet until crisp. Drain on paper towels. Crumble bacon and add to a greased 4–6-quart slow cooker. Brown ground beef in skillet, drain of grease, and add to slow cooker.
- Add remaining ingredients to slow cooker. Cook on high for 4–6 hours or on low for 8–10 hours. Serve with Gluten-Free Corn Bread (see recipe in Chapter 3).

SPICY BEANS AND RICE CASSEROLE

Servings: 8

Ingredients:

- 1 (15-ounce) can whole kernel corn, drained

- 1 (15-ounce) can black beans, rinsed and drained
- 1 (10-ounce) can diced tomatoes with green chilies
- 1 cup brown rice, uncooked

Ingredients:

- 2¼ cups gluten-free chicken broth or water
- 1 cup gluten-free salsa
- 1 cup Cheddar cheese, shredded
- ¼ cup chopped fresh cilantro, for garnish

Directions:

- Grease a 4-quart slow cooker. Add corn, beans, tomatoes, rice, chicken broth or water, and salsa. Cover and cook on high for 3 hours or on low for 6 hours.
- Once rice has absorbed water and is fully cooked, stir in Cheddar cheese. Cook an additional 20 minutes on high to melt cheese, and serve. Garnish with cilantro.

TUSCAN CHICKEN AND WHITE BEANS

Servings: 4

Ingredients:

- **3 large boneless, skinless chicken breasts**
- **1 (15½-ounce) can white beans, drained and rinsed**
- **1 (14½-ounce) can diced tomatoes**
- **1 (4-ounce) can mushrooms, drained**
- **¼ cup Spanish olives stuffed with pimientos, sliced in half**
- **2 teaspoons onion powder**

Ingredients:

- 1 teaspoon garlic powder
- 1 teaspoon basil
- 1 teaspoon oregano
- 1 teaspoon ground pepper
- ½ teaspoon salt
- 2 teaspoons olive oil

Directions:

- Cut chicken breasts into large chunks and place in a greased 4-quart slow cooker.
- Add beans, tomatoes (including the juice), mushrooms, and olives. Add onion powder, garlic powder, basil, oregano, ground pepper, and salt.
- Mix all ingredients together in the slow cooker. Drizzle olive oil over the top of the chicken and vegetables.
- Cook on high for 3½–4 hours or on low for 6

hours. Serve over cooked rice or gluten-free pasta, if desired.

LEMON-GARLIC GREEN BEANS

Servings: 4

Ingredients:

- **1½ pounds fresh green beans, trimmed**
- **3 tablespoons olive oil**
- **3 large shallots, cut into thin wedges**
- **6 cloves garlic, sliced**

Ingredients:

- 1 tablespoon grated lemon zest
- ½ teaspoon salt
- ½ teaspoon pepper
- ½ cup water

Directions:

- Place green beans in a greased 4-quart slow cooker. Add remaining ingredients over the top of the beans.
- Cook on high for 4–6 hours, or on low for 8–10 hours. If you like your beans crisper, check them on high after about 3½ hours or on low after about 6 hours. Fresh green beans are sturdy enough to

withstand very long cooking temperatures without getting mushy.

CLASSIC BEANS AND FRANKS

Servings: 6

Ingredients:

- 1/4 cup onion, finely diced
- 2 teaspoons butter
- 1 (16-ounce) can gluten-free baked beans
- 1 (16-ounce) package gluten-free hot dogs, cut into 1/2" slices

Ingredients:

- 1/3 cup brown sugar
- 1 teaspoon ground mustard
- 1 teaspoon celery salt

Directions:

- In a small glass or microwave-safe bowl, cook onion and butter on high for about 1 minute until onion is soft. Pour into a greased 2 1/2-quart slow cooker.
- Add baked beans, hot dogs, brown sugar, mustard, and celery salt to the onions and mix well.
- Bake for 4 hours on high or for 8 hours on low.

PINTO BEAN-STUFFED PEPPERS

Servings: 4

Ingredients:

- 1 cup cooked rice
- 1 (15-ounce) can pinto beans, drained and rinsed
- 1 (15-ounce) can tomato sauce

Ingredients:

- 1 packet gluten-free taco seasoning
- 4 medium red, yellow, or green peppers

Directions:

- In a large bowl mix together the rice, pinto beans, tomato sauce, and taco seasoning.
- Carefully remove the tops, seeds, and membranes of the peppers. Fill each pepper with 1/4 of the pinto bean mixture.
- Place the stuffed peppers in a greased 4-quart slow cooker. Add 1/3 cup of water around the bottom of the stuffed peppers.
- Cook on high for 3–4 hours or on low for 6–8 hours until peppers are softened.

BARBECUE CHICKEN AND BEANS

Servings: 4

Ingredients:

- 3–4 chicken breasts, cut into 1" pieces
- 1 (14½-ounce) can red kidney beans, drained and rinsed
- 2 teaspoons gluten-free Worcestershire sauce

Ingredients:

- 1 cup gluten-free homemade or store-bought barbecue sauce
- 2 cups cooked white rice

Directions:

- Add all ingredients, except rice, to a greased 2½-quart or larger slow cooker.
- Cook on high for 4 hours or on low for 8 hours. Serve over rice.

BLACK BEAN AND CHEESE TACOS

Servings: 4

Ingredients:

- 1 (15-ounce) can black beans, drained and rinsed
- ¾ cup mild gluten-free salsa
- 8 gluten-free corn taco shells

Ingredients:

- 1 cup shredded Cheddar cheese
- 1 heart of romaine lettuce, shredded

Directions:

- Add black beans and salsa to a greased 2½-quart slow cooker. Cook on high for 3–4 hours or on low for 6–8 hours.
- Fill each taco shell with several tablespoons black bean filling, several tablespoons of shredded cheese, and a handful of shredded lettuce.

THREE BEAN SALAD

Servings: 8

Ingredients:

- 1 (15-ounce) can black beans, thoroughly rinsed and drained
- 1 (15-ounce) can red kidney beans, thoroughly rinsed and drained

- 1 (15-ounce) can chickpeas (garbanzo beans), thoroughly rinsed and drained
- 1 green pepper, finely diced
- 2 medium red onions, finely diced
- 1/3 cup cider vinegar

Ingredients:

- 1/4 cup extra-virgin olive oil
- 1 clove garlic, finely diced
- 1 tablespoon honey
- 1/2 teaspoon ground mustard
- 1/2 teaspoon salt
- 1/2 teaspoon black pepper
- Handful of fresh cilantro, chopped

Directions:

- In a large bowl, mix the black beans, red kidney beans, and chickpeas. Add the diced pepper and onions and mix well.
- In a small bowl, combine the vinegar, oil, garlic, honey, mustard, salt, and black pepper. Once thoroughly mixed, pour over bean mixture.
- Add cilantro and refrigerate for 3–4 hours before serving.

TRICOLOR TOMATO-BEAN SALAD

Servings: 6

Ingredients:

- 3 plum (Roma) tomatoes, seeded and chopped
- 1 green tomato, seeded and chopped
- 1 yellow tomato, seeded and chopped
- 1 small cucumber, peeled and chopped into 1" wedges
- 1 (15-ounce) can small white beans, thoroughly rinsed and drained

Ingredients:

- 1/2 red onion, finely chopped
- 3 tablespoons extra-virgin olive oil
- 2 tablespoons balsamic vinegar
- 2 cloves garlic, crushed
- 1 teaspoon gluten-free Dijon mustard

Directions:

- Place the tomatoes, cucumber, beans, and onion in medium-sized bowl.
- In a small bowl, whisk together the oil, vinegar, garlic, and mustard until completely blended.
- Pour oil and vinegar mixture over chopped

vegetables. Stir to thoroughly combine. Refrigerate for at least 1 hour or overnight.

HEALTHY MEXICAN CASSEROLE

Servings: 8

Ingredients:

- 1 tablespoon extra-virgin olive oil
- 1 pound lean ground turkey
- 1/2 teaspoon cumin
- 1/4 teaspoon gluten-free chili powder
- 1/4 teaspoon red pepper flakes
- 1/8 teaspoon coriander

Ingredients:

- 2 tablespoons water
- 1 (15-ounce) can black beans, rinsed thoroughly and drained
- 1 (15-ounce) can pinto beans, rinsed thoroughly and drained
- 4–5 plum (Roma) tomatoes, chopped and seeds removed
- 1 teaspoon chopped chili peppers
- 1/2 cup frozen corn
- 1/4 cup Mexican blend shredded cheese

Directions:

- Preheat the oven to 350°F.
- Heat the oil in a large skillet over medium-high heat. Cook turkey in hot oil for 5–8 minutes, until the meat is browned.
- Stir in cumin, chili powder, red pepper flakes, coriander, and water.
- Add black and pinto beans, tomatoes, chili peppers, and corn. Stir well.
- Place the meat mixture in a 9" × 13" casserole dish and add cheese on top.
- Bake for 20 minutes until cheese is melted.

THICK AND CREAMY CORN AND BLACK BEAN CASSEROLE

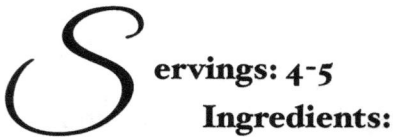

Servings: 4-5
Ingredients:

- **2 tablespoons unsalted butter**
- **½ sweet onion, chopped fine**
- **½ cup minced celery**
- **½ cup minced celeriac (celery root)**
- **¼ cup sweet red pepper, roasted and chopped**
- **2 tablespoons corn flour, potato flour, or cornstarch**
- **½ cup rich gluten-free chicken broth**

- 1 (15-ounce) can black beans, thoroughly rinsed and drained
- 1 (10-ounce) package frozen corn kernels

Ingredients:

- 2 large eggs, well beaten
- 1½ cups whipping cream
- 1 teaspoon salt
- 1 teaspoon sweet paprika
- 1 teaspoon ground black pepper
- 1 teaspoon ground coriander
- ½ teaspoon ground allspice
- 1 cup gluten-free bread crumbs
- 1 cup grated Cheddar cheese

Directions:

- Preheat the oven to 350°F.
- Melt the butter in a large ovenproof casserole. Add the onion, celery, celeriac, and red pepper and sauté over low heat until vegetables are soft, about 10 minutes.
- Mix in the corn flour or starch and stir, cooking gently for 3 minutes.
- Add the chicken broth, black beans, and corn. Bring to a boil, and then lower the heat to a simmer and cook until the black beans are slightly softened, about 20 minutes. Take off the heat.

- In a small bowl, mix together the eggs and cream. Blend the mixture quickly into the vegetables. Mix in the salt and spices.
- Place in a well-buttered casserole or keep in the same ovenproof pan that you've been using for cooking. Sprinkle the top with bread crumbs and cheese.
- Bake until golden brown and bubbling, about 15 minutes. Serve hot.

WARM TOMATO BEAN SALAD

Servings: 4

Ingredients:

- **1 tablespoon grapeseed oil**
- **3 cloves garlic, chopped**
- **1 (15-ounce) can white cannellini beans, rinsed and drained**

Ingredients:

- 5 plum (Roma) tomatoes, chopped
- 1 cup baby spinach

Directions:

- Heat the grapeseed oil in a skillet over medium-high heat, and sauté the garlic for 1–2 minutes,

until soft.
- Pour the beans and chopped tomatoes into the skillet. Reduce heat to medium-low and simmer for 5–10 minutes, until the tomatoes are soft.
- Remove from heat and stir in spinach until wilted.
- Serve over chicken or as a side dish.

FIESTA LIME-LENTIL SALAD

Servings: 8
  Ingredients:

- 1 (16-ounce) bag dried lentils
- 4 cups water
- 1/2 teaspoon sea salt
- 2 tablespoons freshly chopped cilantro
- 1 tablespoon grapeseed oil
- 1/2 cup broccoli, chopped
- 1/4 cup carrots, sliced
- 1/2 cup green cabbage, chopped
- 1/4 cup radish, chopped
- 1/2 green pepper, chopped

Ingredients:

- 1 celery stalk, chopped
- 2 cloves garlic, minced
- 1/4 teaspoon ground chili pepper
- 1/2 teaspoon dried oregano

- 1 teaspoon dried basil
- 1 teaspoon dried cumin
- 1/2 teaspoon dried paprika
- 1/2 teaspoon ground gluten-free cayenne pepper
- Juice of 1 lime

Directions:

- Rinse the lentils under running water and pick through them to remove any bits of soil or rocks.
- Add the lentils and water to a saucepan (with a lid) and bring to a boil. Turn heat down to low and cover to let the lentils simmer, but leave the lid ajar a bit so that they don't boil over. Check on them occasionally to make sure the water has not boiled down below the level of the lentils; add more water as needed. When the lentils are tender and can easily be mashed with a fork, they are done. It usually takes about 30–45 minutes for them to cook.
- Add salt and cilantro in about the last 15 minutes of cooking time—when the lentils are starting to get soft. (Cooking often neutralizes the taste of the salt, so if you add it at the start, you end up having to add more salt to get the same flavor.)
- When they are finished cooking, take the saucepan off the heat and cover tightly with the lid. Let sit for 5–10 minutes. The lentils will absorb more of the water, making them juicier and more tender.

- In a large skillet over medium heat, add the oil and chopped veggies and sauté for 5 minutes.
- Add lentils and seasonings and stir. Let sit on medium-low heat for 5–8 minutes until the veggies soften.
- Remove from heat, add fresh lime juice, and stir until well blended.

QUINOA PILAF WITH LENTILS AND SPINACH

Servings: 4

Ingredients:

- **1 tablespoon butter**
- **½ medium onion, finely chopped**
- **1 clove garlic, minced**
- **½ cup uncooked quinoa, rinsed and drained**
- **1½ cups gluten-free vegetable broth**
- **½ cup uncooked lentils, rinsed and dried**
- **1 tablespoon extra-virgin olive oil**

Ingredients:

- 1 cup water
- 2 carrots, finely chopped
- 1 teaspoon oregano, dried
- 1 teaspoon basil, dried
- 4 cups baby spinach
- Salt and pepper, to taste

- 1/4 cup toasted almonds, for garnish (optional)

Directions:

- Place butter in large skillet over medium heat. Add onion and garlic and cook 3–4 minutes, until onion is translucent.
- Add rinsed quinoa and let sit for 1 minute until brown. Add broth and bring to a boil. Reduce heat, cover, and let simmer on low heat until all broth is absorbed, about 15–20 minutes.
- While quinoa is cooking, place dried lentils and olive oil in a small skillet. Add water, carrots, oregano, and basil. Bring water to slight boil over medium-high heat, then reduce heat to low. Cook lentils for 20–30 minutes, until tender.
- When quinoa is finished cooking, stir in baby spinach. Add salt and pepper.
- Combine lentil mixture and quinoa together. Garnish with toasted almonds if desired.

BLACK BEAN-QUINOA CHILI

Servings: 10

Ingredients:

- **1 cup uncooked red quinoa, rinsed and drained**
- **2 cups gluten-free vegetable broth**

- 1 tablespoon canola oil
- 1 green onion, chopped
- 5 cloves garlic, chopped
- 1 tablespoon gluten-free chili powder
- 1 tablespoon cumin, ground
- 1 teaspoon coriander, ground
- 2 cups plum (Roma) tomatoes, diced
- 2 cans black beans, rinsed and drained
- 1 green bell pepper, chopped

Ingredients:

- 1 jalapeño pepper, seeded and chopped (optional)
- 1 tablespoon dried chipotle pepper
- 1 zucchini, chopped
- 1 teaspoon dried oregano
- 1/2 teaspoon dried cinnamon
- Salt and ground black pepper, to taste
- 1 cup frozen corn
- 1 cup portobello mushrooms, chopped
- 1/4 cup fresh cilantro, chopped
- Sliced avocado, plain gluten-free Greek yogurt, and shredded Cheddar cheese for topping

Directions:

- Place quinoa and broth in a medium saucepan over high heat and bring to a boil. Cover, reduce heat to

- medium-low, and let simmer for 15–20 minutes, until all the broth is absorbed. Set aside.
- Heat oil in a large skillet. Add the onion and garlic, and sauté for 3–4 minutes, until soft. Add the chili powder, cumin, and coriander. Stir to combine.
- Add the tomatoes, beans, peppers, zucchini, oregano, and cinnamon. Mix well and season with salt and pepper.
- Bring to a boil over high heat, reduce to low heat, cover, and let simmer for 20 minutes.
- After 20 minutes, add the quinoa, corn, and mushrooms, and cook for an additional 5 minutes to soften corn and mushrooms. Remove from heat.
- Top with sliced avocado, a dollop of plain Greek yogurt, cilantro, and shredded cheese.

SPICY QUINOA BEAN BURGERS

Servings: 6 burgers
   Ingredients:

- **1/2 cup uncooked quinoa, rinsed and drained**
- **1 cup gluten-free vegetable broth**
- **1 (15-ounce) can black beans, rinsed and drained**
- **1 (15-ounce) can red kidney beans, rinsed and drained**
- **1 cup baby spinach**
- **3/4 cup cornmeal or gluten-free bread crumbs**

- 1/4 cup red bell pepper, chopped
- 1/4 cup frozen corn, defrosted
- 1/4 cup mushrooms, finely diced
- 1 shallot, minced

Ingredients:

- 1 clove garlic, minced
- 1 teaspoon gluten-free chili powder
- 1/2 teaspoon red pepper flakes
- 1 teaspoon cumin
- 1 teaspoon paprika
- 1 teaspoon fresh cilantro, chopped
- 1 teaspoon gluten-free hot sauce
- 1 large egg
- Juice of 1/2 fresh lime
- Fresh avocado slices and tomato slices for topping

Directions:

- Preheat the oven to 375°F.
- Place the quinoa and broth in a small saucepan and bring to a boil. Cover, reduce heat to low, and simmer for 15–20 minutes, until all the broth is absorbed.
- Place the beans and spinach in blender or food processor and process for 1 minute allowing for some pieces of whole beans to remain.
- Place the quinoa in a medium-sized bowl. Add the

beans/spinach mixture, cornmeal, bell pepper, corn, mushrooms, shallot, garlic, seasonings, cilantro, hot sauce, egg, and fresh lime juice. Thoroughly mix with your hands to combine. If you have time, sit bowl in the refrigerator for a few minutes. This allows for easier forming of the patties.

- Form the quinoa/bean mixture into 6 patties. Line baking sheet with aluminum foil and place patties on top. Bake for 30 minutes, making sure to turn them over after first 15 minutes.
- Serve on top of rice or sautéed spinach and top with avocado and tomato slices. You can also eat these burgers with a gluten-free bun or in a gluten-free wrap or wrap each one in a giant lettuce leaf.

SUN-DRIED TOMATO–ARTICHOKE PASTA WITH WHITE BEANS

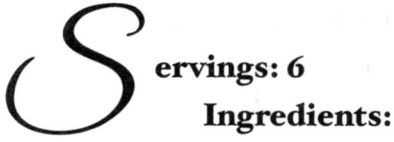

Servings: 6
Ingredients:

- 1 tablespoon grapeseed oil
- 3 cloves garlic, finely chopped
- 1 cup sun-dried tomatoes, sliced
- 2 cups chopped mushrooms

- **1 (9-ounce) box frozen artichoke hearts, rinsed and drained**

Ingredients:

- 1 (15-ounce) can small white beans, rinsed thoroughly and drained
- 2 cups gluten-free vegetable broth
- 3 cups arugula
- 1 (16-ounce) package brown rice pasta
- 2 tablespoons freshly shaved Parmesan cheese (optional)

Directions:

- Place the oil and garlic in large skillet and let simmer for 1–2 minutes, until the garlic softens.
- Add the sun-dried tomatoes, mushrooms, artichoke hearts, and beans, and let simmer for 3–4 minutes, until they soften.
- Add broth and let simmer for 3–4 minutes. Add arugula, mix well, and remove from heat. You do not want the arugula to get too soft.
- Cook the brown rice pasta according to instructions. Rinse pasta with cool water and drain.
- Mix pasta with broth and veggie mixture. Top with shaved Parmesan if desired.

SWEET POTATO AND BLACK BEAN HASH

Servings: 4

Ingredients:

- 2 tablespoons extra-virgin olive oil
- 1 medium onion, thinly sliced
- 2 cloves garlic, minced
- 1 small yellow pepper, chopped
- 2 medium sweet potatoes, peeled and diced into 1/2" cubes
- 1 jalapeño pepper, seeded and minced (optional)
- 1 1/2 teaspoons cumin
- 1 teaspoon coriander

Ingredients:

- 1/8 teaspoon gluten-free cayenne pepper
- 1/2 teaspoon gluten-free chili powder
- 3/4 cup gluten-free vegetable broth
- 1 (15-ounce) can black beans, rinsed thoroughly and drained
- 2 tablespoons fresh cilantro, diced
- Salt and pepper, to taste
- Sliced avocado, lime wedges, diced scallions, and gluten-free sour cream, for garnish (optional)

Directions:

- Heat the olive oil over medium heat in a large skillet. Add onions and garlic and cook for 3–4 minutes.
- Add the yellow pepper and cook another 2 minutes until they all start to brown.
- Add the sweet potatoes and continue to stir while they brown. Cook for another 5 minutes. Add jalapeño pepper (if using), cumin, coriander, cayenne pepper, and chili powder. Stir to combine.
- Add broth and continue to stir for 3–4 minutes, until liquid is absorbed.
- Add beans and continue to stir, making sure everything is completely mixed. Add cilantro, and season with salt and pepper.
- Can be served warm or cold. Garnish with sliced avocado, lime wedges, diced scallions, or sour cream, if desired.

Chapter Six

SNACKS AND DESSERT

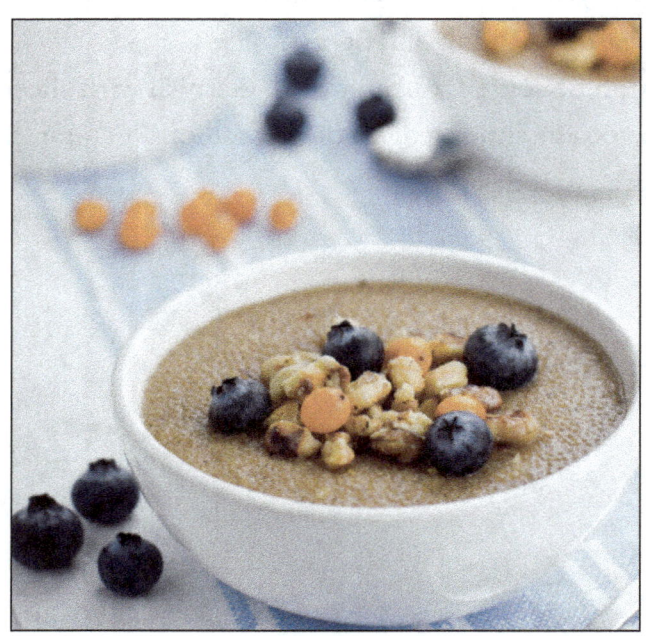

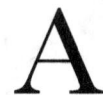vocado-White Bean Hummus

Servings: 10

Ingredients:

- 1 (15-ounce) can cannellini beans, drained and rinsed
- 1 ripe avocado, peeled, pitted, and diced
- 1 large garlic glove, coarsely chopped
- ¼ cup water, plus more as needed
- Juice of 1 lemon

Ingredients:

- 2 tablespoons extra-virgin olive oil
- 1 teaspoon kosher salt
- 2 tablespoons coarsely chopped fresh cilantro
- Freshly ground black pepper

Directions:

- Place the cannellini beans, avocado, garlic, water, lemon juice, olive oil, salt, chopped cilantro, and pepper in a food processor fitted with a blade attachment or a high-speed blender.
- Process until smooth, scraping down the sides of the bowl as needed. If the dip is too thick, pulse in more water, a tablespoon at a time, until the

desired consistency is reached. Serve with Baked Corn Tortilla Chips

BAKED CORN TORTILLA CHIPS

Servings: 6
Ingredients:

- **24 gluten-free corn tortillas**

Ingredients:

- 1 teaspoon kosher salt

Directions:

- Preheat the oven to 350°F.
- Cut tortillas into large triangular slices. Lay slices out in a single layer on a baking sheet and sprinkle with salt.
- Bake 8–12 minutes, or until chips start to lightly brown. Repeat with remaining tortilla slices. Let cool for 10 minutes before eating.

GOLDEN PARMESAN CRISPS

Servings: 12 crisps
Ingredients:

- 2 tablespoons unsalted butter (more if necessary)
- 12 heaping tablespoons coarsely grated fresh Parmesan cheese

Ingredients:

- 1 teaspoon thyme
- Freshly ground black or gluten-free cayenne pepper, to taste

Directions:

- Heat the butter in a large fry pan over medium heat until it bubbles.
- Spoon the cheese by tablespoonfuls onto the butter, pressing down lightly with the back of the spoon to spread, making 12 tablespoon-sized crisps.
- After about 2 minutes, turn and cook until both sides are lightly golden brown. Add more butter if necessary.
- Sprinkle with thyme and black pepper or cayenne, or both. Serve at once.

RASPBERRY YOGURT SMOOTHIE

Servings: 2

Ingredients:

- **INGREDIENTS:**
- **1 cup plain nonfat gluten-free Greek yogurt**
- **½ cup frozen raspberries**
- **½ cup fat-free milk (almond, soy, or milk of your choice)**

Ingredients:

- ½ banana
- 2 tablespoons ground flaxseed

Directions:

- Place all of the ingredients in blender for 1–2 minutes until thoroughly
- blended. Serve immediately.

CHOCOLATE-PEANUT BUTTER SMOOTHIE

Servings: 2

Ingredients:

- **2 tablespoons unsweetened cocoa powder**
- **2 tablespoons natural creamy gluten-free peanut butter**
- **½ banana, frozen**
- **½ cup almond milk (or milk of your choice)**

Ingredients:

- ½ cup plain gluten-free Greek low-fat yogurt
- ½ teaspoon vanilla extract
- 4–5 ice cubes

Directions:

- Combine all ingredients in a blender and blend until thick and creamy.
- Serve immediately.

BLUEBERRY-OATMEAL SMOOTHIE

Servings: 2

Ingredients:

- **½ cup gluten-free rolled oats**
- **1 cup soy milk**
- **1 banana, frozen**

Ingredients:

- ¾ cup fresh or frozen organic blueberries
- 1 teaspoon honey (optional)
- 4–5 ice cubes (if using fresh blueberries)

Directions:

- Place the oats in a blender and blend for 1–2 minutes until they are ground into a fine powder.

- Add the rest of the ingredients, blend, and enjoy!

SNEAKY KIWI-PINEAPPLE SMOOTHIE

Servings: 2 smoothies

Ingredients:

- 1 cup pineapple chunks, fresh or frozen
- 2 kiwis, peeled and chopped
- 1/2 banana
- 6 ounces plain gluten-free Greek yogurt

Ingredients:

- 1/2 cup pineapple juice
- Ice (you can use less if you use frozen pineapple)
- 2 tablespoons chia seed or flaxseed (optional)
- 1 cup spinach or kale (optional)

Directions:

- Place all the ingredients in a blender. Blend until smooth.
- Serve immediately.

MIXED BERRY SMOOTHIE

Servings: 2-3

Ingredients:

- 2 cups unflavored almond milk, or milk of your choice
- 1 tablespoon 100% pure maple syrup
- 1 teaspoon vanilla extract
- 1/2 cup frozen raspberries

Ingredients:

- 1/2 cup frozen strawberries
- 1 tablespoon coconut oil
- 1/2 teaspoon cinnamon
- 1/2 cup blueberries, frozen

Directions:

- Place all ingredients into a blender container in the order listed.
- Blend until smooth, about 1 minute. Pour into glasses and serve.

POPCORN WITH PARMESAN TOPPING

Servings: 8

Ingredients:

- 1 tablespoon grapeseed oil
- 1 cup popcorn kernels

Ingredients:

- 1/2 teaspoon sea salt
- 1/2 cup Parmesan cheese, freshly grated

Directions:

- Place grapeseed oil in bottom of a large pot.
- Place popcorn kernels on top of the oil in the pan. Do not turn stove on yet. Stir kernels to make sure they are evenly coated with the oil.
- Place heat on medium and, with the pot uncovered, shake the kernels around in the pot until the first kernel pops. Quickly place the lid on top and wait until all the kernels pop.
- Once done, remove from heat and add salt and Parmesan cheese. Stir to mix thoroughly. You can store popcorn in an airtight container for up to 6 months.

HOMEMADE SWEET POTATO CHIPS

Servings: 3 dozen chips
Ingredients:

- **2 large sweet potatoes, peeled**
- **3 cups canola oil**

Ingredients:

- Salt and pepper, to taste

- 1 teaspoon cinnamon (optional)

Directions:

- Slice the potatoes thinly with a mandoline.
- Heat the oil in a deep-fat fryer to 375°F.
- Fry potato slices for about 3–4 minutes, depending on the thickness of the chips. When the chips are very crisp, remove from the oil and drain.
- Add salt, pepper, and cinnamon if desired. Serve with a gluten-free dip or eat plain.

APPLE AND PEAR NACHOS

Servings: 4

Ingredients:

- **1 sliced apple, cored**
- **1 sliced pear, seeds and stem removed**
- **2 tablespoons raw almond butter, slightly heated**
- **2 ounces pecans, walnuts, almonds, or nuts of choice**

Ingredients:

- Chocolate chips, to taste
- Golden raisins, to taste
- Shredded coconut

Directions:

- Arrange apple and pear slices on a plate.
- Pour the melted nut butter over the top. Then add nuts, chocolate chips, raisins, coconut, or any other of your favorite toppings, and serve immediately.

PARMESAN-KALE CHIPS

Servings: 6
Ingredients:

- **1 bunch kale (the curly kind is less bitter)**
- **1 tablespoon extra-virgin olive oil in Misto sprayer**

Ingredients:

- 1 teaspoon salt
- 1 tablespoon finely, freshly grated Parmesan cheese

Directions:

- Preheat oven to 350°F. Line a non-insulated cookie sheet with parchment paper.
- With a knife or kitchen shears, carefully remove the kale leaves from the thick stems and tear into bite-sized pieces. Wash and thoroughly dry kale with a salad spinner.

- Spray the kale with olive oil from Misto sprayer and sprinkle with salt and Parmesan.
- Bake until the edges brown, but are not burned, 10–15 minutes.

BANANA-NUTTER SANDWICH

Servings: 6

Ingredients:

- **1 loaf No Grain Bread**
- **½ cup natural gluten-free peanut butter**

Ingredients:

- 3–4 large bananas, sliced

Directions:

- Slice loaf of bread into 12 slices.
- Spread peanut butter on 6 slices, then add sliced bananas.
- Place remaining bread slices on top to make a sandwich.

SWEET CHERRY-QUINOA GRANOLA BARS

Servings: 18 bars

Ingredients:

- **1½ cups gluten-free puffed rice cereal**
- **1 cup pure rolled oats (make sure they are gluten-free)**
- **1 cup cooked quinoa**
- **½ cup gluten-free dried cherries, unsweetened**
- **⅓ cup sunflower seeds**
- **⅓ cup sliced walnuts**
- **¼ cup pumpkin seeds**

Ingredients:

- 2 tablespoons flax, ground
- 2 tablespoons chia seed, ground
- 1 teaspoon ground cinnamon
- ½ teaspoon sea salt
- ⅓ cup sunflower seed butter
- 6 tablespoons 100% pure maple syrup

Directions:

- Preheat the oven to 325°F. Line a baking sheet with parchment paper and set aside.
- In a large mixing bowl, combine all ingredients, except the sunflower seed butter and maple syrup.
- In a small saucepan, heat the sunflower seed butter and syrup over medium low heat until it becomes liquefied and smooth.
- Pour the liquid ingredients over the dry ingredients

and mix together until fully combined and everything is coated evenly.
- Spread the granola out on the parchment-lined baking sheet, into a thin 1/4" layer.
- Bake in the center of a warmed oven for 25 minutes, until the granola is browned and slightly crispy. (Don't cook any longer; it may not look burned but it will be.)
- Let the granola cool for about 10 minutes on the baking sheet.
- Transfer to a flat surface and cut into bars and finish cooling on a wire rack. Enjoy either in bar form or crumble as granola pieces. Store in an airtight container, for up to 5 days.

PEPPERONI PIZZA QUESADILLAS

Servings: 4

Ingredients:

- **8 gluten-free corn or brown rice flour tortillas**
- **2 cups Easy Pizza Sauce , plus extra for dipping**
- **8 ounces shredded mozzarella cheese**

Ingredients:

- 1/3 pound gluten-free pepperoni

- Sliced mushrooms, peppers, onions (optional)

Directions:

- Brush each tortilla with a thin layer of pizza sauce (so thin that if you turned it over, none would drip).
- Sprinkle cheese on top of the sauce on the bottom tortilla. Top with pepperoni and other toppings, if desired. Sprinkle with another layer of cheese and place the other tortilla on top (sauce side in).
- Lay out tortilla and place it on a griddle or in a pan sprayed with cooking spray and cook for 3–5 minutes on each side, until cheese is melted and tortillas are crispy.
- Slice into quarters and serve with a little bowl of pizza dipping sauce.

EASY PIZZA SAUCE

Servings: 2¾ cups

Ingredients:

- 1 teaspoon extra-virgin olive oil
- 1–2 cloves garlic, finely chopped
- ½ medium onion, finely chopped
- 1 (15-ounce) can tomato sauce
- 1 (6-ounce) can tomato paste

Ingredients:

- 1 tablespoon ground oregano
- 1 teaspoon ground basil
- ½ teaspoon turbinado sugar
- ½ teaspoon salt

Directions:

- In a skillet over medium heat, place the oil, garlic, and onions. Simmer until they soften, about 2–3 minutes.
- In a medium bowl, mix together tomato sauce and tomato paste until smooth. Stir in oregano, basil, sugar, and salt. Add the cooked garlic and onions. Makes sauce for about 4 (10") pizzas.

CHOCOLATE MINT SWIRL CHEESECAKE WITH CHOCOLATE NUT CRUST

Servings: 10-12

Ingredients:

- 1½ cups ground walnuts (the food processor works well)

- ½ cup sugar
- ⅓ cup unsalted butter, melted
- 4 ounces semisweet chocolate, melted
- 4 large eggs, separated
- 3 (8-ounce) packages cream cheese (not low- or nonfat)
- 1 cup gluten-free sour cream

Ingredients:

- ¾ cup sugar
- 1½ teaspoons pure vanilla extract
- 1 teaspoon salt
- 2 tablespoons chestnut flour
- 4 ounces semisweet chocolate
- 2 tablespoons peppermint schnapps
- Whipped cream for topping (optional)

Directions:

- In medium bowl, mix the first four ingredients together. Spray a 9" springform pan with nonstick spray and press the walnut mixture into the bottom to make a crust. Chill for at least 1 hour.
- Preheat the oven to 350°F. In a clean bowl, beat the egg whites until stiff. In a separate large bowl, using an electric mixer, beat the cream cheese, sour cream, sugar, vanilla, salt, and chestnut flour. Melt 4 ounces semisweet chocolate with the schnapps.

- With the motor running, add the egg yolks, one at a time, beating vigorously. Fold in the stiff egg whites. Using a knife, swirl the chocolate and schnapps into the bowl.
- Pour into the springform pan and bake for 1 hour. Turn off the oven, and with the door cracked, let the cake cool for another hour. Chill before serving. You can add whipped cream to the top before serving.

CHERRY VANILLA CHEESECAKE WITH WALNUT CRUST

Servings: 10-12

Ingredients:

- 1½ cups ground walnuts
- ½ cup sugar
- ½ cup unsalted butter, melted
- 4 large eggs, separated
- 3 (8-ounce) packages cream cheese

Ingredients:

- 1 cup gluten-free sour cream
- 2 teaspoons pure vanilla extract
- 1 teaspoon salt
- 2 tablespoons rice flour
- ⅔ cup cherry preserves, melted

Directions:

- Mix together the walnuts, sugar, and melted butter. Prepare a springform pan with nonstick spray and press the nut mixture into the bottom to form a crust. Chill for at least 1 hour.
- Preheat oven to 350°F. Beat the egg whites until they form peaks and set aside. In a large bowl, using an electric mixer, beat the cream cheese, sour cream, vanilla, salt, and rice flour together.
- Add the egg yolks, one at a time, while beating. When smooth, fold in the egg whites and mix in the cherry preserves.
- Pour into springform pan and bake for 1 hour. Turn off oven and crack the door. Let cake cool for another hour. Chill before serving.

LEMON CHEESECAKE WITH NUT CRUST

Servings: 10-12

Ingredients:

- 1¼ cups ground walnuts (or whatever nuts you like)
- ½ cup sugar
- ½ cup unsalted butter, melted
- 5 egg whites
- 3 (8-ounce) packages cream cheese
- 1 cup gluten-free sour cream

- 2/3 cup sugar

Ingredients:

- 2 tablespoons rice flour
- 1 teaspoon salt
- 3 egg yolks
- Juice of one lemon
- Minced rind of 1 lemon
- Extra nuts to sprinkle on top of cake, paper-thin lemon slices

Directions:

- Mix together the ground nuts, sugar and melted butter. Use nonstick spray on a springform pan. Press the nut mixture into the bottom to form a crust, and chill.
- Preheat oven to 350°F. Beat the egg whites until stiff and set aside. Using an electric mixer, beat the cheese, sour cream, sugar, flour, salt, and egg yolks, adding the yolks one at a time. Beat in the lemon juice and lemon rind.
- Gently fold in the egg whites. Pour the cheese/lemon mixture into the springform. Bake for 1 hour. Turn off oven and crack the door, letting cool for another hour. Chill before serving. The chopped nuts and thinly sliced lemon add a nice touch.

MOLTEN LAVA DARK CHOCOLATE CAKE

Servings: 8

Ingredients:

- 8 teaspoons butter to grease custard cups
- 8 tablespoons sugar to coat buttered custard cups
- 8 ounces semisweet baking chocolate
- 6 ounces unsalted butter
- 3 large eggs

Ingredients:

- 3 egg yolks
- 1/3 cup sugar
- 1 tablespoon chestnut flour
- 1 teaspoon vanilla
- 1 quart raspberry sorbet

Directions:

- Prepare the insides of 8 (6-ounce) custard cups with butter and sugar. Preheat oven to 425°F. Over very low heat, melt the chocolate and butter in a heavy saucepan.
- In a large bowl, using an electric mixer, beat the eggs, egg yolks, sugar, flour, and vanilla for about 10 minutes. Add the chocolate mixture by the

tablespoonful until the eggs have absorbed some of the chocolate. Fold in the rest of the chocolate/butter mixture.
- Divide the mixture between the custard cups. Place the cups on a cookie sheet and bake for 12–13 minutes. The sides should be puffed and the center very soft. Serve hot with raspberry sorbet spooned into the "craters."

MOLTEN SWEET WHITE CHOCOLATE CAKE

Servings: 8

Ingredients:

- 8 teaspoons butter to grease custard cups
- 8 tablespoons sugar to coat buttered custard cups
- 8 ounces unsweetened white baking chocolate
- 6 ounces unsalted butter
- 3 large eggs
- 3 egg yolks

Ingredients:

- 1/3 cup sugar
- 1 tablespoon chestnut flour
- 1 teaspoon vanilla
- 1/2 teaspoon salt

- 2 cups mixed berries, such as strawberries, raspberries, and blueberries

Directions:

- Prepare the insides of 8 (6-ounce) custard cups with butter and sugar. Preheat oven to 425°F. Melt the chocolate and butter over low heat in a heavy saucepan. In a large bowl, using an electric mixer, beat together the eggs, egg yolks, sugar, and flour. Add vanilla and salt.
- Keep beating and slowly add, by the tablespoonful, 1/4 of the white chocolate mixture. When well blended, add the rest of the chocolate mixture, very slowly.
- Divide between the custard cups, place on a cookie sheet, and bake for about 12 minutes. Serve with mixed berries in the "craters." You can also vary this by using shaved bittersweet chocolate in the craters, or you can spoon in gluten-free ice cream or sorbet.

ORANGE CARROT CAKE

Servings: 8-10

Ingredients:

- **4 large eggs, separated**
- **1/2 cup brown sugar**

- 1½ cups grated carrots
- 1 tablespoon lemon juice
- Grated rind of ½ fresh orange

Ingredients:

- ½ cup corn flour
- 1" fresh gingerroot, peeled and minced
- 1½ teaspoons baking soda
- ½ teaspoon salt

Directions:

- Liberally butter a springform pan and preheat oven to 325°F. Beat the egg whites until stiff and set aside.
- Beat the egg yolks, sugar, and carrots together. Add lemon juice, orange rind, and corn flour. When smooth, add the gingerroot, baking soda, and salt. Gently fold in the egg whites.
- Pour the cake batter into the springform pan and bake for 1 hour. Test by plunging a toothpick into the center of the cake—if the pick comes out clean, the cake is done.

CLASSIC PAVLOVA CAKE

Servings: 6

Ingredients:

- **4 egg whites**
- **1 teaspoon vinegar**
- **4 ounces sugar**
- **1 cup heavy cream**

Ingredients:

- 3 tablespoons confectioners' sugar
- 1/2 teaspoon vanilla
- 1 banana, sliced
- 1 quart strawberries, washed, hulled, and halved, 8 left whole for decoration

Directions:

- Preheat oven to 200°F.
- Whip the egg whites, and as they stiffen, add the vinegar and slowly add the sugar. Pour into a 9" glass pie pan that you've treated with nonstick spray.
- Bake the meringue for 2 hours. Then, turn off the oven and crack the door. Let the meringue rest for another hour. It should become very crisp and lightly browned. Do not store it if the weather is humid.
- Whip the cream and mix in the confectioners' sugar and vanilla. Slice a layer of bananas onto the bottom of the cooled meringue crust. Add a layer

of whipped cream. Sprinkle with halved strawberries.
- Add another layer of whipped cream and decorate with the whole strawberries. Serve immediately or it will get soggy.

CHESTNUT COOKIES

Servings: 48 cookies

Ingredients:

- 1 (2-ounce) can chestnuts, roasted, peeled, and packed in water
- 1½ cups chestnut flour
- ½ cup fat-free milk
- 2 egg yolks
- 1 teaspoon vanilla
- ½ teaspoon nutmeg

Ingredients:

- 1 teaspoon salt
- 2 teaspoons gluten-free baking powder
- ½ cup granulated sugar
- ½ cup unsalted butter, melted
- 3 egg whites, beaten stiff

Directions:

- Preheat the oven to 350°F.
- Drain the chestnuts and chop in the food processor. Place in the bowl of an electric mixer. With the motor on low, add the chestnut flour, milk, egg yolks, vanilla, nutmeg, salt, baking powder, sugar, and melted butter.
- Fold the egg whites into the chestnut mixture. Drop by the teaspoonful on cookie sheets lined with parchment paper.
- Bake for 12–15 minutes. Cool and place on platters for immediate use, or store in tins for later use.

CHOCOLATE MERINGUE AND NUT COOKIES

Servings: 40 cookies
Ingredients:

- **½ cup sugar, divided**
- **¼ cup unsweetened cocoa powder**
- **⅛ teaspoon salt**

Ingredients:

- 3 egg whites (from extra-large eggs)
- ⅛ teaspoon cream of tartar
- ½ cup hazelnuts, lightly toasted, skinned, and coarsely chopped

Directions:

- Preheat oven to 275°F. Line two cookie sheets with parchment paper. Sift 1/4 cup of sugar and 1/4 cup of cocoa together in a bowl. Add salt.
- Beat egg whites with cream of tartar. When peaks begin to form, add the remaining 1/4 cup sugar, a teaspoon at a time. Slowly beat in the cocoa mixture. The meringue should be stiff and shiny.
- Add chopped nuts. Drop by teaspoonfuls on the parchment paper. Bake for 45–50 minutes. Cool on baking sheets. You can place these in an airtight cookie tin or serve them the same day.

APPLE COBBLER WITH CHEDDAR BISCUIT CRUST

Servings: 8-10
Ingredients:

- **2 cups corn flour**
- **1/2 teaspoon salt**
- **4 teaspoons gluten-free baking powder**
- **1/2 teaspoon gluten-free cayenne pepper**
- **1/4 cup margarine, softened**
- **3/4 cup buttermilk**
- **3/4 cup grated sharp Cheddar cheese**
- **8 large tart apples such as Granny Smiths, peeled, cored, and sliced**

Ingredients:

- 1/3 cup lemon juice
- 2 teaspoons cinnamon
- 1/4 teaspoon nutmeg
- 1½ tablespoons cornstarch
- 1/4 cup dark brown sugar
- 1/4 cup white sugar
- Pinch salt
- 4 tablespoons butter

Directions:

- Preheat the oven to 325°F. In a large bowl, mix the flour, salt, baking powder, and pepper. Cut in the margarine with a large fork until it looks like oatmeal. Add the buttermilk and stir. Add the cheese and set aside.
- Place the apples in a large baking dish, about 9" × 13", or a 2-quart casserole. Sprinkle them with lemon juice.
- Mix together the spices, cornstarch, sugars, and salt. Toss the apples with this mixture. Dot with butter. Drop the cheese mixture by the tablespoonful over the top.
- Bake for 50 minutes, or until crust is browned and the apples are bubbling. Serve with extra slices of cheese or with vanilla ice cream.

www.ingramcontent.com/pod-product-compliance
Lightning Source LLC
Chambersburg PA
CBHW070910080526
44589CB00013B/1246